Vasundhara Raghavan retired as general secretary of Mumbaibased Media Research Users Council. She and her husband Srinivas live in Dubai. They have two sons. You can contact the author at v.ramanujan@yahoo.com

Mohammad Akmal is a professor of medicine at the USC Keck School of Medicine and has directed its dialysis programme for more than twenty-five years.

To
People touched by disease: patients, families, and friends

SHADES OF LIFE

SUBLIME JOY IS IN LIVING

How a young man's journey through kidney disease helped his family find meaning in their lives

VASUNDHARA RAGHAVAN,
DR. MOHAMMAD AKMAL

Solomon Trust Media

There is no wealth but life.

—John Ruskin

Table of Contents

Foreword

Aldous Huxley stated, 'Experience is not what happens to you. Experience is what you do with whatever happens to you.'

Not one of us can determine what happens to us. At best we can take actions that improve or reduce probabilities. But when what has to happen, happens. We tend to behave in a pattern—take credit if it is positive, pass the blame if it is not so good.

Vasundhara Raghavan's son was diagnosed with a completely unexpected and serious kidney problem, out of the blue, without warning or time to prepare. She and her family responded, and this is her story: engaging, courageous, positive-spirited and demonstrating that hope is the only way to respond to human difficulty. When a kidney transplant became essential, she marvelled at God's creation, she did not blame Him.

As she writes:

> The human mind has remarkable capacity to observe and store such special incidents in life for recall at an appropriate time. I realised that all this ado was a silent tribute to God, through whom such miracles are possible.

She also reflects on life itself:

> Life is a great mystery. The more we try to solve it, the more we get involved. The situation gets complicated, as we want immediate results. There is no magic formula for achieving our dreams. Everything needs time and patience till we can hit the button to success. Until that time, we must simply permit life to take its course. In that alone will there be peace.

I have been touched by two other books of this genre, *Chasing Daylight* by Eugene O'Kelly and *Does He Know a Mother's Heart?* by Arun Shourie. Vasundhara's work measures up to those books. It is moving and endearing, yet hugely inspirational. The world needs more people who can and will share answers to two questions:

- What happened to me?
- What did I learn from responding?

Mumbai
20 February 2012

R. GOPALAKRISHNAN
Director, Tata Sons

Preface

This book is a reflection of how two people deal with chronic kidney disease—one, a mother who has been taking care of a beloved son affected with kidney failure for a major part of his life, and the other, I, a doctor who has spent most of his life treating such patients.

I have been a kidney specialist for more than thirty years and have had the opportunity not only to provide medical care to a diverse group of patients with various kidney problems, but also to be an active participant in volunteer services through the National Kidney Foundation. Aditya began studying at the University of Southern California (USC), and hence became my patient. When I first met Aditya's mother, Vasundhara, I was immensely impressed with how devoted and keenly interested she was in her son's medical problems. She not only helped Aditya cope with kidney failure, which meant dialysis and related limitations, dietary restrictions, and compliance with medications, but was also a great motivator who helped him continue his education with enthusiasm and dedication. While he was at the University, she visited him regularly from Dubai so that his educational activities did not falter and that he religiously adhered to his medical regimen.

My co-author's honesty, integrity, emotional stability, positive and outgoing attitude, sociability, trustworthiness and self-confidence set her apart from most other people. My respect for her began with our first meeting and continued to grow as I got to know her while I was her son's physician. It was interesting that we shared many values, including our children's education. My two sons were undergraduate students at the USC, where Aditya, then a postgraduate student, and his brother, both also studied. I have also been serving at the science campus of the University for more than thirty years. My two sons are now medical doctors, and Aditya is a doctor of philosophy. The friendship and cohesiveness between Vasundhara and me is built on our care for Aditya, to whom she donated one of her kidneys, which lasted several years. We share a common goal: to participate in activities that could help millions of people who suffer from kidney failure.

Finally, I am impressed with Vasundhara's intelligence and writing ability, which exudes personal emotions and is based on her own experiences. I am proud to be her partner in writing this book and the series of books that will follow.

25 November 2009

MOHAMMAD AKMAL, MD
Professor of Medicine
Keck School of Medicine
University of Southern California

Introduction

Ihad the chance to be associated with kidney disease twice before my fiftieth year. The first time, it involved my friend Malathi. We were barely ten years old, so my understanding of the disease was very limited. All I could make out was that it had simply led to instant death. The death of a dear friend at an impressionable age was a great blow. The killer disease, which gradually attacked and destroyed five of the seven children in that family, was mystifying. This was in 1962, when treatment for this disease was probably unheard of in Bombay (Mumbai),

India's commercial capital.

As I grew up, the unhappy memory of my friend receded. I bounced back to life, enjoyed my youth, entered womanhood, settled into marriage, and looked forward to 'magical happiness' ever after. Very soon reality hit me; I learned that life was a journey of challenges. It made good sense to confront them as they surfaced.

But my life's experiences had done little to prepare me to meet the second episode of kidney disease, the one that changed the way I breathed. My son was stricken by this disease.

I asked myself then, 'Why should I presume that it would be different for others?'

While embarking on a cure for this killer disease, I gathered a lot of valuable information. With the singular purpose of spreading this information, I became serious about writing a book about my journey through this disease. February 2004 saw the birth of *Shades of Life: Sublime Joy Is In Living.* The concept was good, the sentiments even better, but it was extremely difficult to put pen to paper to write about the harsh facts of life.

But the purpose was not to entertain, but to inform.

Reminding myself every day about what I was here to deliver, I worked my way through the book. It could help kidney patients to understand the enormity of the disease, be better prepared to meet the ordeal, find a solution to a life-threatening problem, and find a way to save their kidney. Reports from most countries in the world shows conclusive evidence that many adults are at risk of losing their kidney functions. Not many are aware that they are below the radar.

Low awareness is seen as the primary factor leading to increasing incidence of end-stage renal failure among individuals within certain demographic parameters such as age, sex, ethnicity, education, and medical conditions like hypertension. In some cases, awareness could be preventive; in others, it can be curative; and there will be some for whom it will mean a lifetime of health care. The hope that people will be able to live, and continue to enjoy life, is the fine print.

I hope my family's story will give the reader reason to lead life with awareness and sensitivity.

I read somewhere that life is a great big canvas on which one can paint one's dreams and see them blossom. The basic sketch gets a frame where events of the day are captured with pencil marks. Finally, with many more sketches, a complex picture of a person's life emerges. There are some grid lines, fitted with intricate lines to make this picture a good, realistic portrait: simple, smooth, thin lines depict fun and happiness, reflecting cheerfulness and flamboyance. Sharp, thick lines mark difficult periods of sorrow, failures, and hardships. Vibrant colours add to the hue and complement the drawing. Different shades of colour bring the portrait to life.

This is what life is, I surmised—a fine portrait, and each one is different from the other. None of them are better or worse, as there is equal opportunity for each one to be a winner.

The portrait is as alive as it can be. It has flesh. Red blood flows through it. The heart beats. Love and laughter express joy. Songs are sung. Anger shakes the form and figure. And so we live on, with all expressions and emotions embedded in the portrait.

The portrait needs to be preserved till the end, as it is ordained. Every effort is needed to keep it safe and nurture it with utmost love and care. It is the life of a human being that we are preserving.

The picture of life is painted by one, but due to the intense and close interactions between many people who directly or indirectly influence our lives, the etchings are sometimes darker and deeper. If one were to step aside and study the painting, it would be tempting to erase some of those dark, ugly lines.

But the journey through life is one template that cannot be modified. This understanding shaped *Shades of Life: Joy Is In Living*.

Dubai   VASUNDHARA RAGHAVAN
25 November 2009

First Signs

28 November 1996

It was the winter of 1996. Lovers of cricket in India were in raptures because the country's team had defeated the visitors from South Africa. Other than the volume of news from radio, television, and the press, it was the outbursts in my living room from my nearly seventeen-year-old son Dhananjay and his brother, Aditya, a year and half younger, that most often engaged my attention. Both of them were ardent cricket lovers who spent time discussing and statistically analysing the game. I loved the boisterous hullabaloo that floated through the open drawing room, dining area, and kitchen, mingling with the noise and flavours of my burning hearth.

My husband, Srini (also known as Srinivas Raghavan), worked as a senior engineering professional in the petroleum and gas agency. Our family was happy and content and I beamed with joy at the thought.

But my joy was short-lived as I was troubled by another thought. Aditya had missed school for two days. His complaint was a headache. As a questioning parent, I wondered if he was not facing up to the reality of his Class Ten examinations looming large or if it was truly something in the brain area.

On day three, when the headache persisted, I called my office, asking for a few hours' absence, and we went immediately to meet Dr Manda, our family physician. I narrated the incidents of the past few days—about Aditya's constant headache which was not relieved even after the consumption of a variety of pain relievers. She examined him, the back side of her palm on his temple and surprisingly, along with her stethoscope, she pulled out the instrument to check his blood pressure. After rechecking, she summoned her superior. For a third time, they checked Aditya's blood pressure.

The doctors' expressions bordered on amazement.

I braced myself to question them. The senior doctor spoke hesitatingly; she sensed a problem, as the blood pressure was high for a fifteen-and-a-half-year-old. She suggested a blood test to identify the problem. The doctor called the pathologist at Doctor House, asked for an urgent appointment, and placed a request for an intermediary analysis report.

In two hours, the preliminary test results were spread on her table, and she studied them carefully. Looking up, she said, 'It's surprising, the creatinine level is very high.'

Taking a deep breath, and looking for some support from her junior, the doctor said, 'I believe there could be some problem with the kidneys.'

As we looked on, surprised at what she had said, she continued, 'You should get this checked with a specialist.

Dr Bhupendra Gandhi, attached to Breach Candy Hospital is a very experienced, senior doctor. He will be able to guide you.'

She scribbled a short note to the doctor and told us that the doctor was available during the clinic's evening hour. It would be appropriate to visit him at six o'clock in the evening.

Entering the Hospital Gates

28 November 1996

The impressive white structure of the Breach Candy Hospital nestles on South Mumbai's west coast, with rocks guarding it from the Arabian Sea's acts of violence. On normal days, the sea-facing rooms in the hospital enjoy the view of water lashing against the boulders and then flowing down gracefully in submission. Rough weather

predictably influences the sea's tumultuous mood.

This visual drama provides a backdrop to run away with one's thoughts, thoughts that are sometimes peaceful and at other times serious contemplations on life.

The hospital, over decades of service to the human race, has established itself as an institution with proven medical talent, offering world-class health care and diagnostics. Treatments and surgeries requiring high-precision skills and expertise are conducted here by well-reputed doctors who contribute to making this place a choice for people seeking, among other things, high standards of hygiene and cleanliness.

Since the hospital generally attracts patients with deep pockets, we were worried about how we could be financially affected if we required the hospital's services in the future. We took directions from the reception staff to the kidney centre. Stepping out of the elevator, we were surprised to hear noise and merriment. Then we realised that, since it was the visitors' hour, the paediatric ward had a happy atmosphere created by the merry chatter of families and friends, celebrating the arrival of a newborn.

In no particular mood to participate, we turned our attention to finding the long, pale-green-walled corridor that would lead us to the operating theatre. We found the corridor, where whiffs of the strong, acrid smells of disinfectants touched our senses. This area needed the toughest armour against infections. Halfway down, another corridor on the left sent us straight to our destination.

Though we had had the opportunity to visit the hospital before, that occasion had not involved personal medical consultations. We walked with apprehension as uncertainty about Aditya's health and the severity of his illness weighed heavily on our minds. As a headache was a simple, everyday ailment, we wondered why much ado was being made about it. Relying on our doctor's advice on a subject of which we had little knowledge, we decided to try to understand how a headache could bear relation to a kidney problem.

A tough façade, but totally traumatised inside, could describe how we presented ourselves at the nurse's table with our doctor's introductory note. We waited in the lobby with other people, some of who gave a knowing look. We chose to keep our counsel and wait with patience, acquired with difficulty.

The doctor greeted us with a smile as we entered his chamber. Unsure of how to introduce ourselves, I blurted out Aditya's condition— the nagging headache, the visit to an optometrist, and the medical examination by the family doctor, with no positive result. The discomfort had persisted. Dr Bhupendra Gandhi proved to be a man of few words.

He checked Aditya's blood pressure, studied the blood test report, made some notes, repeated the blood pressure check, and shared his preliminary observations by analysing it for us. He said, 'Some things need to be seen.'

After a brief pause he continued, 'From the blood report it appears that his creatinine is high . . . the normal range is

0.6 to 1.2 mg/dl, but in this case . . . Aditya's . . . it is 4.58 mg/dl, which is rather high.' We waited with bated breath, our eyes watching him closely. His eyes were on the report, his fingers busy feeling the texture of the paperweight placed on it.

'The level of potassium at 5.9 mg/dl is also on the higher side, and, considering he is a young man, a little over fifteen years old, I am afraid his blood pressure, at 140/90, is not normal. I would say it is rather high.'

We remained quiet.

He continued in a plain voice, 'It looks like Aditya has some kidney-related problem. Some tests are needed to confirm the exact condition. Only after full investigation can we be sure.'

There was silence from all of us. It was broken when he cleared his throat and, picking up his letter pad, scribbled orders for tests, including Complete Blood Count (CBC), Blood Urea Nitrogen (BUN), ultrasound sonography, and abdomen X-ray.

Anxiety prompted me to ask questions to clear up my doubts as they surfaced, 'Doctor, if this is a kidney problem, will it mean dialysis?'

As if giving it some thought, the doctor responded slowly, 'It is possible that he would need that,' and then, when I probed further whether a transplant was a possibility, he added cautiously with his eyebrows arched, 'Yes, even a transplant could be on the cards, but it is still very early to comment.' Pointing to the document in his hands, he added, 'You know, we need to do all these tests before anything can be confirmed.'

He spoke comfortingly, adding that every effort would be made to treat the condition through diet and mild medication.

After nodding our consent to do the tests, we left his chamber feeling totally lost. I don't know how we scrambled out of the hospital, but we knew that getting home immediately would bring relief.

It is difficult to maintain sanity when one hears of a very serious health condition. There is confusion. Thinking is clouded by doubt. Someone should objectively break through the brain cells to speak out loud: 'Go slow; think with your head, not your heart; do not get swayed by emotions; be dispassionate. Try to quell all waves of emotion that could destroy sanity and an opportunity to do it right.' Driving home, I checked with Aditya on his reactions.

Shrugging his shoulders in a matter of fact manner, he said, 'I don't know, Amma . . . it's so sudden.'

After a while he spoke, adopting a different tone, 'But you know, what is there to doubt . . . such an experienced doctor certainly will know what he is saying . . . no chance that he will be making some random statement.'

As soon as we entered the safety of our home, my first reaction was to inform my husband. Srini was required to travel outstation for client meetings and to go to construction sites, and sometimes he was even directly involved with project construction and execution. Currently he was involved with some projects being executed in Baroda, a city of the second greatest economic significance in the state of Gujarat, and he had been away for the past four days.

I called him at his workplace.

Slowly, as my news registered, Srini responded in monosyllables, taking in details as I incoherently broke down the information.

'Srini, remember Aditya was complaining about a headache? So, we went to Dr Manda. Imagine, she checked his blood pressure, Dr Shah also checked it, and it turned out to be rather high, and on the basis of that she asked us to get his blood tests done! So we rushed to Doctor House, and the pathology department did the test, and the doctors found his creatinine to be very high.'

Quite taken aback, Srini kept probing, 'Are you sure? It is surprising . . . hmm . . . what was the creatinine level?'

'Around 4.5 mg. The normal level is something like 0.6 to 1.2 mg/dl. Just a few minutes back, we returned from Breach Candy Hospital. We met a nephrologist, Dr Bhupendra Gandhi. He is in charge of the hospital's dialysis centre, and he is an expert in the field. He suspects it to be a kidney failure of some sort. Tomorrow we need to do some tests—sonography and X-ray.'

Finally the news seemed to hit Srini, and he spoke with barely masked anxiety, 'Are you saying Aditya has a kidney failure?'

Attempting to be in control of the situation, I simply added, 'I don't know how, Srini, but the doctor seemed so sure. I believe he is right. Somehow both Aditya and I feel that this . . . this could be it.'

'I see . . . let us do the tests tomorrow and see. But this is bad news,' he added in his characteristic manner. I could sense his nervousness and shock. 'I will be back tomorrow morning.'

The rest of the evening I found Aditya quiet and thoughtful. He was sometimes worried, sometimes sad and questioning and at other times doubtful about what his life would be. I thought of the many unexpressed desires of an adolescent, which he would never be able to talk about. In a sudden sweep, the very meaning of life was changing for him.

Investigation and Diagnosis

30 November 19962

The tests were important, so without any further questioning, we got straight into the act.

With the doctor's prescription in hand, we reached Breach Candy as early as possible, aiming to manage the time between tests efficiently so all the results would be ready the same evening. We would meet Dr Gandhi at six o'clock. After giving blood samples at pathology for the CBC and BUN tests, we moved to the radiography section for the sonography and the abdomen X-ray. Dr Gandhi had mentioned that the ultrasound sonography of the kidneys

would help in locating the problem.

The radiologist asked us a few basic questions on Aditya's health conditions and a brief family history. A technician applied some lubricating gel on Aditya's abdomen. She spoke gently, asking him to relax, since the procedure was not painful.

The procedure started, with the transducer slowly moving across his abdomen, relaying faint images on the screen, which we could not decipher. She moved it around for a while, exerting some pressure near the area where the kidneys were situated. She pointed out to us the right kidney and then the left, showing the exact area where the kidneys had shrunk in size due to repeated infections. She remarked that the condition of the right kidney seemed quite bad.

Her assessment prepared us for what to expect when we met the doctor later that day. It is the doctor who would finally reveal the truth and explain the extent of the kidney's damage. We awaited his verdict.

Srini joined us for our evening meeting with Dr Gandhi. The wonderful thing about Srini was his ability to think logically and analytically. With use of these capabilities, understanding facts and making clearer decisions would be possible.

Dr Gandhi studied the results of all the tests.

From the X-ray and sonography reports, he pointed to the exact location of the problem. In layman's terms, he explained, 'The right valve is defective, so some urine which should normally come out from the bladder is going back to the kidney. There is a reverse flow of urine.'

Leading us to a dummy anatomy of the renal system that stood on a side table, with his hands gliding across it, he began explaining, 'Here, this is the right valve. Normally it opens only downward so the urine from the kidney goes into the bladder and then through the urethra it goes out of the body. But when this valve is defective, as in Aditya's case, the valve swings forward and backward freely, so when the bladder is full, the urine is waiting to leave the bladder, but the fullness of the bladder builds up extreme pressure, leading to partial reverse flow of the urine into the kidney. Over several years this backflow has infected the kidney.'

He rechecked Aditya's blood pressure, and then he moved his hand upward from Aditya's ankle to his thigh, checking for any abnormal swelling. 'Swelling means water retention, which is a bad sign. Aditya would require Lasix to remove the excess body fluids.'

After taking a pause to gather his thoughts, the doctor informed us that Aditya's kidneys were gradually heading toward complete failure. They were presently functioning partially, but this condition would last only for a short time. Much depended on how well we managed the kidneys' condition.

With his forehead creasing slightly, Srini questioned, 'Doctor, why do you think this happened?'

Gandhi explained that it was a congenital problem—a condition that was present at birth. It might not necessarily be a genetic problem. It is a condition known as vesicoureteral reflux, and it was at Grade IV stage. In its final stage, Grade V, both the urethra and the kidney would be severely affected, while the pelvis and the calyces would be extremely dilated.

He added, 'This would ultimately lead to irreversible chronic kidney failure . . . technically it is called ESRD or End-Stage Renal Disease.'

'Doctor, normally how long does it take to reach the stage of . . end stage?'

'It really depends on how well the medicines work for Aditya. Also, if he is strict with his diet, progression can be controlled.'

After some time, he concluded, 'This damaged kidney condition has resulted in high blood pressure, which caused him the headache, but we have still some time before that stage. Unfortunately, if we had noticed it a few years back, a minor surgery would have solved it.'

Aditya read out the sonography findings, 'Right kidney is 8.3 cm and the left is 8.5 cm. So, Doctor what were their sizes before?'

Turning his full attention to Aditya for the first time, with a smile lighting up his face, the doctor responded, 'The normal kidney size is about 11 cm, almost the size of a fist.' Raising his right fist, he showed it to Aditya to make his point. The doctor was pleased that the young man had opened up.

I observed them and realised with some surprise how this moment would lay the foundation for the doctor- patient relationship. My mind escaped from the environs of the hospital with fleeting thoughts on life. Aditya was ill, seriously ill. These were the harsh facts.

I never dreamed that my teenage son would suffer from one of the world's irreversible ailments. It hurt me deeply to think how close Aditya was to finishing school, and suddenly this boulder had hit us so hard! For him to excel in the board examination meant a few months of dedicated work. It was a crucial period, with projects submission, practical laboratory work, and set deadlines to be met, all needing concentrated effort.

Thereafter, his group at school would be moving out for the first time into an adult world, which was waiting for them to explore and enjoy. It would be time to choose colleges and consider career options, plan a future, and, of course, also date young girls. This was the best time in any young man's life.

All these years I had worried endlessly about Aditya's easygoing attitude. I troubled my mind with unworthy speculations that if he continued to take life lightly, his performance on his final examinations would be poor, and he would be a loser with no career options available. After all, entry into the choicest undergraduate courses was determined by good marks.

Dhananjay, on the other hand, had a serious disposition, was very determined, a deep thinker, and a voracious reader. He had got excellent grades in school, so he was pursuing his undergraduation in his choice of courses. He had also set his goals on following his father's footsteps, though his interest was in electrical engineering, where the world was heading with full gusto.

Aditya loved life. His interests were different. He was a kitchen person, pottering around trying out new recipes. Surprisingly, everything he cooked tasted good. He secretly harboured the desire for a career in hotel management, but the idea was still in its infancy. The family knew he would excel in the hospitality industry, since he had a wonderful way with people of all ages, whom he charmed as he went along.

When he was twelve, Aditya had even experimented with baking bread rolls with wholewheat, using a recipe that called for white flour. He had no particular fancy for reading and serious study was definitely not his forte. So this had been a huge area of concern. The two days he had skipped school to watch the televised cricket match was at the cost of study. Would he make it to the tough outside world with responsibility and bring glory to himself?

The brothers were poles apart, one boisterous and experimental and the other serious and focused. They shared cricket mania, and their food choices were influenced by one another's. The two always seemed to compete for the same things, but, surprisingly, as they grew up, at unexpected times they bonded well. That challenged me in my parenting.

At times Aditya's not gaining height had also worried me. But today neither his physical attributes nor his attitude had anything to do with my pulse racing. My only concern was the huge medical problem that could not be swept under the carpet. It was no longer a straight case.

Suddenly my mind floated back to the hospital room with the doctor and Srini discussing, while Aditya was the quiet spectator. They were talking of medicines for lowering the blood pressure. 'This will be needed over a long period; everything depends on how the blood pressure is controlled also through diet.'

Aditya was thoughtful.

From the subtle change in Srini's face, I realised that he had grown tense. It was difficult to handle a situation like this. I did not know what to do: behave normally, i.e., smile and thank the doctor, or react like many other mothers would in a similar situation—simply cry.

The doctor handed us a prescription for blood-pressure medicines that would help in relieving Aditya of his headache. After some casual talk about Aditya's studies and where my husband worked, we returned home to embrace our new life with the fresh set of problems.

During our drive back home, I noticed that Aditya was quiet. I never got around to asking him what was going on in his mind. As parents, we had to first learn how to handle the situation without losing a grip on the lives of the four of us.

When we reached home, Srini explained the case to Dhananjay and to my mother-in-law.

Dhananjay was quick with questions. He asked, 'So how come we never knew anything before? Do you mean this happens suddenly?'

Srini repeated what the doctor had said about it being congenital. But Dhananjay was not to be easily quelled, so he lashed out, 'What is the treatment for this? Only blood- pressure tablets?'

Even as Srini tried to calm him down and respond as clearly as possible, I realised that Dhananjay's questioning was an expression of his deep sense of hurt. It came out in spurts of anger and tension. He hated to know that his kid brother was being drawn into an adult world, as kidney failure seemed unreal for kids of their age. Guys cannot express this as girls do, I surmised.

His own preoccupation with preparation for his semifinal examinations prior to completion of high school, along with thoughts of college admissions, fuelled his anger—or call it anguish—as he was short on time and energy.

Srini fielded Dhananjay's questions and finally, as if we were waiting for some direction, Dhananjay said, 'Don't you think we should get another opinion? I don't think we can just start Aditya on dialysis. We need to be sure.'

Srini said thoughtfully, 'Yes, I think so.' I knew it was not putting an end to a conversation, but rather clinching our first decision for Aditya's health care.

Aditya was silent all through this animated conversation, letting his dad take the heat. His face wore an expression of reluctance, but he agreed with the family's decision.

The news was gradually conveyed to other family members. Everyone had similar reactions, and we tried to respond to them about matters that were still baffling us.

Questions sprang up in my mind: *Is this curable? Will we be able to resolve this problem? What will be Aditya's future?* I was bogged down by such anxious thoughts, while Aditya too sought answers to many more questions. His was the bigger loss! Although he kept a straight face, not permitting any emotion to surface, deep down, he probably wanted to explode.

We reflected on what the doctor had said: 'The treatment advised will postpone the transplant by several years. It depends on how well you control further damage through proper diet and medication for bringing down the blood pressure.' This put a huge responsibility on our shoulders for getting it right!

He had talked of some patients who had braved this illness with a strict diet that postponed dialysis by seven or eight years. All that was required was a protein-restricted diet, low in salt and potassium.

The doctor had spoken casually, explaining that most human beings were lucky to have two kidneys, when one kidney was sufficient to do the blood purification. By design, the second one was a spare organ and was almost redundant, till a renal failure occurred. This bit of physiology reminded me of what I had studied in school.

Dialysis was the next treatment that might be required when the creatinine levels became very high. At that stage, dietary restrictions alone could no longer control the pace of damage.

Transplant was the last and best treatment, as it gave patients opportunity for a good quality of life.

Reflections

I realised that the doctor could not give us any more comfort or courage.

In his years of work, how many different kinds of patients must have come to him for treatment? Different levels of seriousness, differing attitudes, but possibly similar diagnosis. Sensitising each patient within his or her comfort zone was one of the challenges of his work.

He was very human and sensitive. He suffered the pain that each of his patients experienced. Outwardly, he pretended to be indifferent. As a human, he wanted his patients to walk the path with confidence. That gave him the courage to lead his patients to safety.

Breaking Rules

4 December 1996

In the first few days after Aditya's illness was diagnosed, we could not sufficiently comprehend the complexities of his health condition. As if to give us respite, we were suddenly drawn into the joyous celebrations of a dear friend's daughter's wedding ceremony.

The wedding ceremony was very memorable. I told Aditya casually to watch what he ate. The rest of the evening was spent enjoying the grandeur of the wedding, admiring the parade of beautiful women dressed to the hilt in designer attire, the glitter of gold, gems and stones set on heavy jewellery and the colourful ambience created by floral decorations and the twinkle of lights. All this, topped with melodious music from the shehanai, contributed to the aura of a dream world.

There was an excellent buffet with dishes hand-selected by my friend, representing cuisines from different parts of the world. The spread was so complete that it left little chance for anyone to stay hungry that night. Attempting to be a nonintrusive mother, I hesitantly asked Aditya whether he had enjoyed himself.

He told me in a quiet voice, brimming with excitement, 'I hogged the best of the paneer tikkas; I also had the yummy naan with butter melting from the sides, yumm, yumm. Amma, the samosas were awesome. I enjoyed the chhole- bhatura, it was masaledar (spicy); the Manchurian with the thick soya-sauce gravy was superb. Dhananjay passed me a spring roll. It was nice. Both of us shared a crispy cheese dosa, we tasted the pani-puri, and wow, the dahi-puri simply melted in my mouth. It was super!'

He had visited all the food counters, not leaving out the most delicious malai kulfi, a dip into a hot-fudge nut sundae, desserts, and the fruit platters, including watermelon juice in a tall glass! He had consumed an excessive amount of food, and, to top it all, many of those items were a taboo on the diet list handed out at the hospital just the day before. With a twinkle in his eye, he said, 'Amma, I can never eat such stuff ever again! I did not want to miss this wonderful opportunity.' Dhananjay looked at me in anticipation, his smile guiltless and his eyes barely concealing his anguish.

He knew Aditya would have great difficulty in following a renal diet.

Aditya showed me time and again his love for life and good food. I let the incident pass as an occasion very memorable to him, since he had had the audacity to break all the rules to give himself a huge treat!

Taking the Reins

That Aditya's kidneys were not functioning to their capacity was a reality. Our parental role could at best help Aditya find his chance of living, notwithstanding the health disadvantage. To him our emotions and deep concern were of little consequence. Through strategic thinking, we wanted to devise plans for overcoming problems that he would face, with appropriate actions to offset them.

For centuries humans have always found ways to conquer the world beyond, never letting the thought of failure hold them back. That gave us the impetus to tread territory already covered by many people, with reasonable hope of relief.

The ingredient to achievement was recognising an issue squarely, knowing its depth and dimension, and making calculated decisions to find solutions. In so doing, timeliness is of great significance.

With determination, we lit the flame of hope to sustain us through this phase of life. Our family spent days of unrest, realising that achieving our goal depended largely on our first breakthrough.

We searched for means to steer our lives through the mire. The topic came up at odd times, and it was most often Srini and Aditya who were participants, delving deeper to find information that could guide us. Aditya was never too young to join in the conversation that had great bearing on his life. There was no time to get into sensitivities.

Since maintenance was the first of the three routes for treatment, we looked at the feasibility of maintaining the kidney's condition through diet. For a young person it would be very difficult to enjoy life with food restrictions. The joy of life came through consuming wholesome meals, cooked with salt, enriched with nuts and enhanced flavours to suit the palate. It was ironical that Aditya, who loved food so much that he wanted to join the hotel industry to work on his passion, would now have to forego the pleasures of his taste buds. It was clear to us that for survival such desires would have to be curtailed to match the renal diet that research studies had determined was most suitable for a kidney patient.

So the first change would be in our lifestyle.

The doctor had advised us to meet the hospital dietician for a diet plan. The young medical officer studied the reports and read out some guidelines for Aditya's daily diet. She spoke to us about how food must be cooked with no salt or very little salt. It could be seasoned at the dinner table with a dash of salt. If the food was spicy, the salt content would become higher, so we should limit the use of spices. We should avoid all processed foods, like packaged noodles, ketchup and sauces, including pickles and chutneys, which have hidden salts or sodium.

One small cup of cooked lentils (dal) could be consumed at any one meal in a day. Raw vegetables should be avoided. Greens like spinach were to be avoided, since the blood tests revealed high potassium content. Occasionally a small portion might be consumed. Vegetables were to be leached (double boiled, excess water drained). This would lower the ill effects of excess potassium. For non-vegetarians, fish and meat, which has good-quality protein, might be consumed in small portions, but red meat should be avoided. Fruits such as apples and pears needed to be stewed and consumed in small portions, only occasionally. There was a limit on fluid consumption; it should not exceed two litres. The fluid included water, soups, tea, fruit juice, soft drinks, ice cream and any other liquid. If salt was reduced, consumption of water would automatically be curtailed.

In the case of a renal-failure patient, the diet is based on certain nutritive values. There should be an overall plan to have meals to meet the daily nutrition requirements. Certain food items should be avoided, some could be eaten occasionally, and some others, like carbohydrates such as rice, could form a slightly larger portion of a meal. (Over the years the renal diet devised earlier has undergone change. Research has enabled dieticians to give specific food options for each condition, offering greater flexibility in meal plans.) Our goal was to maintain creatinine at the current level as long as possible, for which Aditya should follow the diet restriction. This would help in postponing dialysis and transplant by a few years.

Apart from the diet, the nephrologists prescribed medicines for bringing down the blood pressure and maintaining it, lowering the level of phosphorus and the absorption of calcium from the gastrointestinal tract, and providing relief against acidity.

Periodic blood-pressure check-ups were also advised. Any time Aditya experienced uneasiness, the first thing he should control is any untoward change in his blood pressure. If there was a rise in BP, he should proactively plan a salt- free lunch or dinner. He could also consult the doctor so that medication for blood pressure could be adjusted. Monthly blood tests should be scheduled to monitor the movements in Blood Urea Nitrogen (BUN), creatinine, and potassium.

We recognised and accepted the first set of action points for health care.

Learning about Kidneys

Our singular purpose was to see that Aditya had the right perspective on his illness. We thought he should fight back and find space in this world. We studied everything related to chronic kidney failure and ESRD with an open mind. With the limited information available to us, we had to get into the finer details about how his health condition would affect his life.

The doctor had explained briefly Aditya's condition. But as more questions crossed our minds, we began our search for information from encyclopaedias and the Internet.

At some time or the other we had seen pictures of kidneys. They are bean-shaped organs the size of a fist, found in the middle of the back, one on each side of the spine. Our only association with the kidneys was that they produce urine by purifying the blood.

But we suddenly became aware that if the kidneys do not work efficiently, normal life will be threatened. We were surprised to know that while most people are born with two kidneys, some people are born with only one.

By chance we came upon knowledge about kidneys that surprised us.

It was news that the kidneys play a major role in maintaining a fit body. They adjust levels of fluids, chemicals, potassium and acids in the body. A person consuming food with excessive salt feels thirsty and tends to consume more water. Under normal circumstances, there is no problem. All the excess will be removed from the body through urine. The body works so silently that we do not notice all the processes that are performed every second.

But if the kidneys fail to function, the patient could be metaphorically 'on the edge of a cliff', with his or her life in danger.

Excess water or chemicals cannot be removed when the kidneys function only partially. Water and wastes harmful to the body build up and remain till they can   be removed.

When kidneys are unable to do all their functions properly, it is called kidney failure.

After the heart and brain, the kidneys are probably the third most important organ, on whose function a person's survival rests.

With our newfound knowledge came a major realisation: that the kidneys' function is underplayed. This was the first-cut information.

Now we had to probe further, sifting through many different bits of information, searching for those crucial for a patient and his or her family.

Information on dangers and pitfalls emerged. We were shocked by the knowledge that water retention could even lead to emergency conditions; all this while we had believed that a diuretic could resolve the condition. In severe cases, even diuretics could not do the trick. Srini also read medical cases of people on dialysis who could not survive the harshness of the treatment. Some people with diabetes already felt challenged controlling their blood sugar through diet; with kidney disease, more limitations were placed, making the diet too restrictive. Patients unable to comply with these diet restrictions faced chances of complications. Yet another group of patients faced consequences due to their non-compliance with medicines and treatments. As for transplants, it was a matter of crossmatch, post-operative care and medical compliance. We read, discussed and debated the side effects of medicines and the details of surgery.

Since we had to negotiate open potholes and danger zones, it was important to hold our ground and mark territories of safety or danger. It was time to sit, plan and execute a plan for survival. We had to accept this as a challenge.

Our main focus was to show Aditya what were the things he must avoid, and what was absolutely necessary and could not be compromised. If he did land in a discomfort zone, we taught him how to escape from that situation.

Aditya was a good learner. Very soon he came out with more things to watch out for. This kept us satisfied, as we were all on the same track without difference in viewpoints. At odd times I caught my mind playing with me. What if Aditya faced such a dire situation? This thought would cloud my thinking suddenly. But with assumed confidence, I would firmly knock down such fears. Though these were random instances, it was a reality for those people who,sadly, were targets of the phenomena. They had not understood clearly how much their health was compromised, or they faced consequences due to other exigencies, or they were unfortunate to be hit, as these things creep up stealthily without an announcement.

We decided what we should do for now: just maintain the kidney condition.

When we reached the stage of dialysis or transplant, we would be ready mentally to handle that eventuality. With basic information, we set the framework and the personal targets for treatment and survival.

The single point of our agenda was to see that Aditya was comfortable.

This was the age and generation when people survived with dialysis and transplants. We should use every such opportunity for our benefit. There was no reasonable excuse for us to default. Taking this stand, we went to find the road to survival.

Establishing a Routine

January to March 1997

On 2 January, we brought home our first blood-pressure unit and stethoscope. It was the old tried and tested mercury meter. After the initial excitement of learning how to use it, we left it to Aditya to learn to examine his own blood pressure.

With regular check-ups becoming mandatory for Aditya, we worked out a schedule for monthly blood tests. It was convenient to do blood tests on the first Thursday of every month. We would meet the doctor with the report the same evening. To ensure that the results were comparable, we decided to do all the tests at Breach Candy Hospital's laboratories.

Aditya's blood-pressure readings were high, with the systolic—the higher level—at 140 and the diastolic—the lower level—at 90.

Aditya's friend Shruti Tandan was studying to be a doctor. She was capable and intelligent and thorough in her work. Effectively using her knowledge and her understanding of Aditya's temperament, she was able to reach out to him at all times. She discussed problems with Aditya as they cropped up. Her book knowledge and field experience were valuable, since she understood the nuances of the disease. Shruti played the crucial role of an in-house doctor. We took the renal diet programme seriously and planned meals around the dietary restrictions. Dhananjay stood by as we reworked dinner menus to suit Aditya's condition. Many food items that Aditya enjoyed were taboo. Cheese and eggs were eliminated from our breakfast table, we used lentils in very limited portions, we avoided processed food and we no longer ordered tomato ketchup and sauces, so French fries, if ever cooked (made with leached potatoes as per renal diet), were not served with any condiments.

Aditya appeared to enjoy even the saltless curries and vegetables, which we leached and then cooked lightly with some basic spices. We experimented with new recipes and combinations of spices, so that Aditya could manage his meals and feel satisfied at the same time. Aditya was a very good patient. He smiled and made me feel less guilty, though I strongly believed the meals were not palatable.

It was a few months before I realised that I had also put Dhananjay on a forced regime, which was not nutritious for a growing young man. I corrected this and began cooking two types of meals—one in line with Aditya's treatment and the other that was suitable for the rest of us.

Gradually we embraced this new lifestyle.

Reflections

Kidney failure leads to a complete change in life for the patient and the family.

The renal diet has so many restrictions that a patient finds it difficult to adopt it. It takes time and an attitude adjustment to accept the diet and understand that change is necessary to find a chance for survival and possibly an opportunity to live longer.

Aditya's daily schedule was crammed with activities. It was a busy period. On the one hand, my capabilities as the key manager of Aditya's health care and diet were being tested, while on the other hand, Aditya and Dhananjay were involved in critical examinations that would chart their life's pursuits. The next few months flew past without any major problems.

I analysed my own actions critically and labelled myself a heartless mom for expecting Aditya to work diligently in preparing for his final examinations (ICSE) without for a moment wondering if he felt tired or had a headache. For fear that my emotional display might cause distraction, I refrained from asking him health-related questions. This guilt weighed heavily on my mind, however.

It was about this time that the British Council Library withdrew a book on renal transplantation, which was supposedly outdated. Srini would read aloud extracts from this hardbound book, which had become a household bible. Aditya would refer to it periodically. He would tell me new things each day. He gathered information from the Internet and would discuss with his dad and Dhananjay details of the chemical compositions of drugs, their side effects, and so on.

Overnight he had grown into an adult. I watched this development with sadness.

My carefree child was now a man of the world, trying to find the means to stay alive. For the rest of his life he would have a heavy burden to carry.

During a doctor's visit, we were alone in the lobby of the kidney centre. It was empty; patients had left for the day. Aditya and I sneaked into the dialysis room. A friendly technician caught us red-handed. He willingly showed us around, explained briefly how the machines functioned, talked about the importance of monitoring weight, and showed us the nurses' station.

Aditya stood there quietly; he probably wondered how it would feel doing dialysis. Such moments were tough for him. I left him to handle his emotions, as this was the natural extension of a lifestyle that would be an integral part of his future.

Time is needed for a person to prepare himself to face a serious illness, with its accompanying challenges. That time was available, since Aditya was diagnosed when creatinine was 4.5 mg, while the stage of dialysis was expected when creatinine bordered around 10-11 mg. At that point, his kidney function would be negligible.

Initially we were in doubt when Aditya's blood pressure rose sharply, leading to a headache. There were times when medication could not bring relief. We questioned our capabilities. But on checking with the doctor, we realised that these issues were part of his health situation. This paved the way for a close association with the doctor, and we sought his guidance whenever it was needed. He was very supportive, and this helped us handle situations better.

Exploring Other Options

Though we were trying hard to accept that Aditya had kidney failure, very early Dhananjay's outburst had told us the value of a second opinion. Knowledge of the gravity of the disease also became reason for confirming whether this was Aditya's health condition. It was too serious a condition to be taken lightly. Taking the lead from some valued suggestions from other family members, we opened our minds to receiving information on alternative therapies.

We decided to leave no stone unturned before concluding what was best for Aditya.

Recognising how critical it would be to handle the disease carefully, the master plan we devised had some basic parameters cast in stone.

The treatment should be medically proven, tried, and tested. A transplant surgery was sensitive, requiring a good hospital with hygienic conditions, capable nephrologists, and an equally competent urologist performing the surgery. The deal-breaker was the post-operative care. The surgery could have after-effects needing urgent medical attention, so hospitals known to offer these services were ranked higher. Having established mandatory conditions, we were confident of reasonable success if we followed our plan to the dot.

Our meeting with several senior urologists and nephrologists in Mumbai confirmed that Aditya's health condition had been diagnosed rightly and that his kidneys were indeed failing. A young doctor was very keen to take us down the corridor to the operation theatre for a preemptive surgery. In his opinion, a young person should not be put through the pain of dialysis. Fear of losing our wisdom and judgement in making an ill-considered decision made us rule out his suggestion.

We took a trip to Nadiad's Muljibhai Patel Urological hospital, located forty kilometres from Ahmedabad. This hospital was gaining prominence as a premier kidney hospital in Gujarat, where organ transplants were conducted in large numbers at very economical costs. The Nadiad Kidney Hospital attracted many top nephrologists and surgeons from across the world, on call for both consultation and surgery.

Considering the logistics of getting there in an emergency when similar facilities were available at some Mumbai hospitals at comparable costs, helped us decide to seek treatment closer to home. Family members made repeated recommendations that we should seek advice from Dr Mani at Chennai's Apollo Hospital. He had rich experience in this field. But we ruled out any treatment outside Mumbai. In order to see if alternative therapies like homoeopathy,

Ayurveda, and Unani could offer Aditya anything, we did some basic checks. Many cases of people cured through these therapies were making news. We assessed popular theories for their strengths and applicability. The cost of treatments was lower, with minimal side effects. Kidney ailments like kidney stones and other types of diseases had been treated successfully.

To initiate our investigation, we tried some Ayurvedic medicines and concoctions and, to a limited extent, introduced Aditya to homeopathic medicines. But we did not pursue these treatments because of our underlying fear of his losing an opportunity to survive.

The sum of all our secondary investigations led us to the conclusion that an experienced doctor with a conservative outlook, whose counselling would be based on established practices for surgery, should be our mentor. The whole episode should not be a roller-coaster ride, as Aditya had a full life ahead.

Aditya made his decision. He chose Dr Gandhi, with treatment at Breach Candy Hospital. His evaluation of the doctor's capabilities in such a short time surprised us.

We accepted his decision.

Reflections

Our goal was to provide Aditya with treatment for a life- threatening disease. If we wavered between therapies, he could lose an opportunity to survive. That was unacceptable. It was important for Aditya to be comfortable with the treatment that we strived to provide him. We were not confident about experimenting on a subject with which we were not conversant. Aditya's knowledge of his health condition made us rely largely on his decision. He was convinced that dialysis and transplant were the best course of treatment.

After all, his life and survival were most important to him.

The Revelation

April 1997

It was in the first week of April that we met a reputed urologist. He remarked that a minor surgery done a few years back could have corrected the problem. During our early meetings, Dr Gandhi had also mentioned this. The kidney could have been saved if the reflux had been detected earlier. In trying to organise our lives under the new circumstance, we pushed the doctor's remark into the darkest recess of our brains.

Now I felt the urgency to know where we had missed the wood for the trees. So we searched wide for what caused renal reflux, which was as Dr Gandhi had explained. It could be a congenital problem for some children due to improper development of the valve when the child was still in the womb.

But this partial information was not helpful, so we searched for the symptoms of reflux. We learned that reflux could be revealed by indications such as urinary tract infection, pain in the back or abdomen, frequent passing of urine or increased passing of urine, bed-wetting, a burning sensation during urinating, the feeling of incomplete emptying of the bladder, and blood in the urine or dark or foamy urine, showing the presence of albumin in the urine.

And, there it was, staring us in the face. Bed-wetting. . . .

This point was lost somewhere in the crowded streets of Mumbai; in the heaps of paper on an unkempt office desk, in a mind that was conquered by an emotional heart. But it was finally unearthed.

An important point and we had not explored it any further! In our naivety, had we been shy of admitting it, of talking about it openly, or guilty of causing too much pain to our dear son?

Very early on, Dr Gandhi had asked us about problems that Aditya faced. With some embarrassment, we had told him about the regular bed-wetting episodes. The doctor had confirmed that this was a consequence of the reflux. For over ten years, we had been troubled by this phenomenon. That Aditya continued to wet his bed after he was six years old had been very disturbing.

I knew of moments of embarrassment that Aditya faced as a kid, especially when he had night-over parties with friends. We would make it light for him and make him feel better. As concerned parents, when Aditya was twelve years old, we had consulted a urologist. After a physical examination, he had remarked that the problem would get resolved when Aditya attained puberty.

As a sibling sharing a room, Dhananjay had been discomforted by these incidents each night. All this was something we bore patiently, assuming that time would heal this condition.

But now my single streak of hope remained in the past: how I wished that I had done something! My motherly instinct should have guided me. A second medical opinion on bed-wetting habits, some essential medical tests, and the problem would have probably been located. Aditya's kidneys would have been saved. He would have been a carefree youngster and loved life even more.

With a very heavy heart, I began an online search for any information on bed-wetting. By chance I clicked on a site that made me sit up and notice. I was not prepared to see it in black and white, but there it was, answering every question that had been raised in my mind. I read with my mouth closed, but unuttered words kept forming in my mouth: 'It is a myth that all children pass urine in bed because they are lazy to go to the toilet. In most cases, bed-wetting is not due to a mental or learning problem. In many cases, bed- wetting is due to what is medically called "enuresis".'

I continued to read, even as I felt the hollowness in my stomach, that kids should get toilet-trained when they are around four years old. If bed-wetting persists after that, a competent doctor must be approached for medical advice. Sometimes bed-wetting may be related to urinary infection. Though bed-wetting may or may not be due to a kidney problem, after a certain age it should not be taken lightly.

It dawned on me that it was certainly in the parents' interest to check with the doctor about whether any medical treatment was required. The website talked of treatments that included repeated urine cultures, with careful monitoring thereafter, antibiotics for infection, ultrasound on an annual basis to monitor developments, and in severe cases, if it is diagnosed in time, treatment through a minor surgery. The surgery could be a ureteral reimplantation or reconstructive repair. Except in rare cases, the problem will not recur.

Finally, the fact stood out as stark reality.

Of all adults and children with reflux, about twenty per cent would end up with renal failure. Such a minuscule percentage of the total world population, yet Aditya belonged here, definitely cordoned off with a tag that read, 'for kidney failure'.

A missed chance need not be mourned, or felt guilty about, but it certainly makes one feel sad. At the end of the tunnel was that door, sealed tight, refusing people their chance to escape.

For a few months I was consumed with emotion, a deep sense of fear and a chilling tremor that shook my insides. My dreams were strange, incomprehensible. I saw a family out there in an open space surrounded by trees, a night that was starless, with no moon to comfort them and no wind whispering through the thick foliage of trees that stood as testimony to their woes. I had visions of a woman clad in a simple white saree, draped tightly around her body, with her husband seated to her left with a face stoic and expressionless, while two young boys were seated, one to her right and the other just facing her. There was pin-drop silence, but the noiselessness was nerve-shattering.

Feeling a huge tremor, their arms flung out and they held on to each other while also desperately holding on to anything to help them survive. Their faces were pale with shock and fear. The woman's eyes rolled upward, beseechingly. Her body twisted with agony and pain, her hands clasped in prayer, her face mournful, asking for mercy, please. . . .

The air hung with strange suspense. Will we make it? Or will we . . . ?

These flashes came even when I was wide awake, my stomach churning under the influence of such absurd dreams. I knew the woman was in deep anguish. A sudden feeling of loneliness and uncertainty engulfed her. And then the prayer that brought momentary calm.

In her I saw a reflection of my own feelings.

A parent—a mother—goes through so many different emotions, but what surfaces is extreme sadness. This goes for every parent whose child is afflicted with a serious ailment. There is life out there, but with many conditions. One needs to brave it, accept some bitter truths, and prepare for a long, rough path ahead. Darkness lurks around the corner. But the mother must prepare her child to take up the challenge and conquer the world. It is a Herculean task, but the child has little option.

I came to accept that the opportunity to give my son a normal life had been lost. I cannot remember any incident that hit me as hard a blow as facing this reality. There could never be another realisation that could shake me to the core or have as much impact.

My moments alone never passed without feeling an insurmountable loss, the kind that only people placed in a similar situation can experience and understand. It took a while to come to terms with, and ultimately acknowledge, that time never rolled back for anyone.

Reflections

The knowledge that early detection could have rectified Aditya's reflux brought another dimension to our thinking. There was enough reason for me to write about the importance of treating urinary infections appropriately with proper monitoring and follow-ups with tests. For bed- wetting beyond age four, there is no reason to delay in seeking medical advice. For that matter, it is also important to control blood pressure and diabetes that could otherwise result in kidney failure.

One should not lose an opportunity to get bed-wetting medically treated. I could not shout loud enough from the tallest high- rise building in this wide world to emphasise this point.

I would say, no one needs to go into that space, where living is treacherous and not meant for universal experience. But one can definitely take measures to safeguard against this condition, since from ESRD there is no return to normalcy. The cost of medical treatment for reflux and urinary infection is small, compared with dialysis and transplant.

The seriousness of kidney failure is difficult to fathom. With each passing day, one notices new challenges. Each issue thereafter has two faces—one of recovery and the other a threat to life.

Reaching each new stage of the disease—enduring the pain of dialysis or managing a transplant—became a reason for sharing this knowledge. If someone catches the early signs, gets help, and uses the opportunity to reverse a case likely to end in a kidney failure, it would be worthwhile. An opportunity to save another kidney, another life, should not be lost.

Parents' roles should include being attentive to a child's needs and being good listeners. As parents we have an important role in talking to, instructing and teaching our child. But, above all, we need to cultivate the art of listening. The child may have a story to tell.

In our busy, urban lifestyle, quality time spent with the kid is a luxury for any parent, particularly in households with working mothers. But this is at the cost of missing an opportunity to find answers to a problem that a child is facing. The problem could be emotional or physical. Sensitivity to the needs of kids should be of prime concern to any parent.

My contribution to the development of my sons was significant. I was conscious of my parental role and made every attempt to excel in it. My waking hours were directed towards developing their inherent skills. I made time for the two boys and learned to enjoy their kind of movies (*Star Wars, Superman,* etc.). I tried living in a boy's fantasy world of camps and tents, vastly different from a girl's world of dolls and playhouses that was part of my childhood. Yet somewhere I had missed that little word or act that would have given me a clue to a problem that lay just below the surface. The clue that would have made a world of difference to my son!

Testing for Tissue Match

12 May 1997

Every meeting with the doctor gave us new tasks, lifting us emotionally and taking us to the next level in decision-making. Our action-list grew with each day. From the day Aditya first asked the doctor a question on kidney size, the relationship between the two of them had blossomed. The doctor discussed with him the medical aspects of blood pressure and medications and how they reacted, and guided him along in keeping his health under control. But every time he discussed Aditya's career plans, he boosted Aditya's ego. That made me cheerful.

During one visit, the doctor broached the subject of a transplant. He advised us to start planning and find a donor. Since Srini is a diabetic, and Dhananjay was still completing high school, the family designated my kidney for donation. The doctor agreed and gave us a prescription for an HLA (a human lymphocyte antigens test) and a crossmatch test.

I took an appointment with Dr Trikannad, an immunologist at Jaslok Hospital. This was another prominent hospital in South Mumbai that boasts of being medically well-equipped with the latest diagnostics and top-level professionals. Samples of blood from both Aditya and me were collected for this test.

The human lymphocyte antigens test is tissue typing, essential for almost all organ transplants. This test would ensure that there was a close match of tissues or cells between the donor and the recipient so that the donated organ would be accepted well. The HLA identifies proteins determined by a particular type of gene within the chromosomes.

The crossmatch is different from tissue-type or blood- group match. Crossmatch is a blood test to check for the existence of any antibodies. Antibodies normally help the body fight infection and would react with the donor kidney. High levels of antibodies may lead to rejection, even if it is a good tissue-type match.

Crossmatch is done by mixing a sample of the recipient's blood with cells from the donor. If your blood starts attacking the donor cells, there is the likelihood of the kidney being rejected.

Our test showed a crossmatch of ten per cent. Above twenty per cent was positive and below twenty per cent was negative.

Dr Gandhi gave a preliminary approval of my kidney for transplant. He mentioned that the match would be higher in the case of siblings.

We were greatly relieved, as Aditya's low-protein, low- salt diet was making life cheerless for the family.

A Twist in the Tale

15 May 1997

Barely two days after Dr Gandhi approved my kidney for transplant, we were in for another surprise.

The family had a relaxed evening after the finding that the tissue match was favourable. The transplant plans had injected some fresh hope in our lives. But by the end of the evening, I lost my cheer as I noticed something unusual— one of my breasts was not as soft as the other. It was hard, and I thought I felt a lump. After some speculation, I conveyed my observation to Srini.

By now it had become normal in our household to discuss illnesses and medical issues. Srini casually suggested that I should get a medical check-up done.

Next morning found me at the Breach Candy Hospital, waiting for an appointment with Dr Jusawalla. This illustrious doctor had gained his reputation by spearheading the opening of the oncology department at Mumbai's premier TATA Memorial Hospital. At this hospital, cancer treatment had become a reality for India, and patients travelled to Mumbai seeking Dr Jusawalla's expert advice. I decided that it should be none other than him to determine my condition, since I was all set to donate my kidney   to Aditya.

The renowned doctor met me along with his protégé, Dr Arun Kurkure.

Dr Jusawalla examined me and confirmed that there was a big, lemon size lump in the upper breast. The doctor was surprised that I had not noticed this earlier through physical examination. I explained my mental state during the past six months. Our family had just managed to get our lives organised under a new lifestyle regime, with our younger son diagnosed with ESRD. Life was not normal anymore.

So many issues had kept my mind occupied that I had not observed any change in my body.

The doctors nodded, with some understanding of my predicament. My explanation seemed tenable to them.

They recommended more tests, and I made appointments with the pathology and oncology departments.

I kept Dr Gandhi informed about, and involved with, these new developments.

The test results confirmed that the lump was significantly large. During discussions the doctors revealed that malignancy of the tumour could only be ascertained during the surgery. On my way home, my mind replayed the conversation with the doctor; I was now more confused than ever. The doctor had said, 'The earlier the surgery is done the better as that will stop further spread.' The doctors had given me tentative dates for the surgery.

Everything was happening so rapidly, there was no time to think. The information filtered in fast, but there was little time to absorb it and react to this situation. It came as an unexpected, unwelcome visitor at my door, on whom it could not be shut.

I realised that my cancer was ill-timed. Our goals were fixed, and with each day we had seen some positive movement towards realising them. Just when we believed some semblance of normalcy was returning to our lives, we were again at crossroads. It was as if we were thrown back into the deep, dark ocean. Would we float or sink? Could we regain our position of strength? This question played in my mind though, outwardly, I seemed relaxed and undisturbed.

Srini felt increasingly weighed down. From a financial standpoint, he was shouldering most of the financial burden resulting from the grave health problems of two members of his family. Though I was in a senior position, my employment in an NGO made my financial contribution to the family's resource pool less significant. He wore his responsibilities on his sleeve, looking to find solutions and finances. He had to balance life, with all its uncertainty, keep the family strong and together, to face the adverse conditions and overcome the hurdles that threatened to sabotage Aditya's health recovery plans.

The boys were surprised, but without a point of view.

Nobody had anything to say.

For Aditya it may have been a sense of disappointment, too. His dream for an early transplant seemed to recede and his early recovery of kidney functions seemed unreal.

At work I held a prominent position with responsibilities in the areas of marketing and administration, and I reported directly to several directors on the company's board as well as to my immediate superior. I informed them of the surgery and took leave.

Reflections

We spend our whole lives trying to find happiness. During the process, we lose an opportunity to enjoy life.

A problem, a potentially fatal medical problem, shakes us inside out. Then there is no time to search for happiness. We discover joy in merely finding remedies to the problems that need attention and solution.

Will we find this joy that evades us? Is there any real joy, or is it a figment of our imagination?

How will we learn to cherish the gift of life and accept its uncertainties? Did we ask for too much happiness, that now we are experiencing this downslide?

And then it struck as lightning . . .

This is God's role—to help us find the way to stay alive and happy.

As we plough through life, we must simply accept that there will be some rough patches that need special attention. As difficult as it gets, we must let destiny take its shape. That does not absolve us of the responsibility for developing the mental capacity to seek happiness and peace.

Mastectomy

30 May 1997

I went into surgery on 30 May 1997 at Breach Candy Hospital. The cancer was at stage II. It was good that we had detected it early. Dr Kurkure did the surgery. Dr Jusawalla and Dr Gandhi were both there. The tumour was metastatic and had spread far and wide, affecting the nodes. A mastectomy was conducted.

Dr Kurkure informed me that a tissue from the infected part had been sent for a biopsy to check for malignancy. At first I knew him to be Dr Jusawalla's assistant, but by the time I finished my surgery, he had masterminded a plan to win my confidence, and I placed my life in his able care.

The remarkable composure Dr Kurkure exhibited showed the value of patience as an important ingredient in a patient's recovery. It remained the single greatest motivating factor in my health care. In his eyes I could see determination to restore my well-being and prepare me for further treatments.

My newfound confidence worked well for both the doctor and the patient.

Later, when Dr Gandhi visited me, I broached the subject of the transplant, which had been on my mind for some time, but the doctor smilingly comforted me, saying, 'It is now crucial for you to get well, you know. Your health is important.'

'But doctor, before the cancer spreads farther, at least the kidney can be transplanted,' I said limply.

The doctor shook his head and said, 'You know, Aditya could be adversely affected if even one cancerous cell got into his system through the transplanted kidney, so you must get fully cured and fit before we could even think of any such surgery.'

Seeing my disappointment, he added, 'There is a very good chance for your full recovery. Today, for treatment of breast cancer, medical science is at a very advanced stage, with high success rates. It is possible that medication will make you fit to be a donor. But for now, take care and get cured.'

He left me very encouraged.

The oncologist had advised me to exercise regularly to get back full vigour and energy. I chose to spend an hour walking on the hospital's terrace.

One evening, Dhananjay visited me early, before other visitors arrived. We walked on the hospital terrace and chatted about things at home. He said his high school examination results were due two days later.

Suddenly getting serious, he said, 'Amma, I think it is better for me not to seek admission at any outstation engineering school. I would like to donate my kidney to Aditya and stay with you at home.'

'Dhanan, I had a chat this morning with Dr Gandhi about the transplant,' I reassured him. 'He says that the treatment for breast cancer is so advanced that there will be a full recovery. Today, survival rates are very high. So don't worry so much. He even said I could donate my kidney afterward.'

Then, on a more serious note, I told him, 'It is important for us to see at least one child go ahead and take up a career of his choice. Do it, Dhanan. Appa and I will be so happy.' The conversation seemed to give him some relief. Smiling with some composure he said, 'Amma, you know, in spite of his headaches, Aditya has done so well. I think it is remarkable. I was doubtful because of his headaches and the sudden health setback. It is really very creditable. I am sure he will get admission into a college of his choice.'

I smiled, patted him on the back, and said, 'Of course, both of you will do well.'

My discussion with Dr Gandhi had given me renewed hope and encouragement. I could respond to my son satisfactorily and help him plan his future.

Reflections

I was very disturbed after my conversation with Dhananjay. There was a huge challenge ahead of us. A small headache that got diagnosed as renal failure came into our awareness at the end of November 1996 and had now grown into a serious disease at such a fast pace.

We had still not got a handle on how to sort out the renal failure, when suddenly we were submerged under another medical problem.

The kids were on the brink of an important period of their lives, where they faced career options, and had to only make crucial choices. Both of them had performed well academically. If their progress was halted, it would not be for lack of effort. My mastectomy had disrupted our plans. I prayed. I wanted us to be back in a position of strength.

Enter the 'Survivors Street', with kidney transplant in the number one slot on the family's agenda. After being discharged from the hospital, I occupied myself with my health care while keeping a watch on Aditya's health. I kept my schedule of weekly visits and check-ups, while he visited the doctor every month. Dr Kurkure advised me on the next treatment. The biopsy report had confirmed that the tumour was malignant. I had to undergo both chemotherapy and radiations.

As my office was running on a skeleton staff, I felt obliged to return early. Twenty days after the surgery, I got permission to rejoin my office, working on a flexible schedule. Thirty days after surgery, I declared myself fit and resumed working full days.

This early return to my desk was a great boon. I noticed Aditya seemingly grow stronger seeing me back in action. I prayed that he should always be in action, in spite of all the odds.

Six sittings of chemotherapy followed by six sessions of radiation were planned. The chemotherapy was done at BCH. The gap between two doses of the chemo was three weeks. By July 1997, I had completed two sessions, and the side effects of the treatment manifested through hair loss. Though I covered my head with a scarf and then later with a wig, evening walks became difficult.

Information on the dos and don'ts during chemotherapy, shared by my cousin Vyu, who had ovarian cancer, was useful. I did the minimum that was required in terms of taking precautions. I had heard that wheatgrass treatment helped reduce the ill effects of chemotherapy. I picked up a bottle of wheatgerm supplements from the health store and added it to my breakfast tray.

By the end of November, I managed to complete my chemotherapy. Many patients were unable to complete the treatment due to their weak constitutions and lowered stamina. The adverse effects of chemotherapy made them vulnerable, especially if they were advised to take a higher dosage. Treatment is different for each kind of cancer and also depends largely on the stage at which it is detected and the rate at which it is spreading.

Between December 1997 and March 1998, the radiation treatment was also completed.

Reflections

The journey through cancer and recovery placed some very harsh facts before me. There were so many millions of people from various strata of society who were caught by the fangs of this dreaded disease. Cancer afflicted them, filling them with pain and worry.

Through this dark phase, hope is a strong light that helps them fight the disease, as almost everyone desires to live.

At the hospital I saw many patients waiting to be treated, but very few machines available and a shortage of technically competent people to do a perfect job—all this in the city of Mumbai, with a vast population of over sixteen million.

I often wondered how many of the patients managed financially. Loud accusations about the treatment and the doctors were heard in many a corridor. These outbursts were an expression of the anguish the patients experienced while battling this most dreaded of illnesses.

I asked myself what was in store for my family and me. I did not wait for an answer.

I did not want to be held in shackles by the fear of the unknown.

I turned my complete will and attention to what needed to be done next.

43

Hugging Life with Dialysis

30 April 1998

Aditya's creatinine levels were gradually increasing. That was a signal of what we could expect.

From November 199€ to November 1997, spanning a period of one year, the creatinine level had shot up from 4.58 mg to 7.€ mg. Within a month of my finishing my radiation treatment, in April 1998, the result of a blood test showed the creatinine at 10.3 mg. This was expected, since on reaching a particular level, the rise is exponential. The kidney had now lost 90-95 per cent of its function and was unable to produce quality urine. The waste products were not getting released from the body. The time to start dialysis had arrived.

Dr Gandhi was travelling. The visiting nephrologists advised us to prepare Aditya for the treatment.

Our own understanding of dialysis was simple. It was a treatment that removed waste products and toxic substances accumulated in the blood, when the kidneys' function was not normal. The treatment would bring Aditya relief. A machine known as the dialyser would play the kidneys' role during dialysis.

Aditya was advised to undergo haemodialysis, which was the more popular treatment. This was done under medical supervision, unlike peritoneal dialysis, which is done by the patient at home and is seen as more convenient. In countries like the United States and Australia, home dialysis is now recommended to patients because of its lower cost.

As a first step, an access, known as a 'fistula', had to be fitted. Aditya had an access put in his right wrist after an hour-long surgery and was discharged the same day. Since the fistula would become operative only after a few weeks, a temporary access was created.

Aditya had his first haemodialysis on 30 April 1998.

The Breach Candy dialysis centre had eight units, and three schedules of dialysis were performed. Aditya wanted to do dialysis here since it had fewer patients. In this environment of quiet and peace, the social interactions would be limited.

He chose the afternoon slot with thrice-a-week dialysis. On the very first day a set of dos and don'ts were handed over. Diet would continue to be restricted.

Haemodialysis, with the tubes of blood flowing outside the body, generally shocks people. Aditya did not show any signs of anxiety. I think he wanted it to be done with so that he could return home feeling better. Before every dialysis, Aditya's weight was measured, which was the wet weight, as there was water in his system, accumulated since the last dialysis. After the dialysis, the weight was again measured. This was the dry weight (weight immediately after the last dialysis). The difference between the wet weight and the last session's dry weight would be the weight gained due to fluid intake and food consumption. If the net weight is high, it may be concluded that the fluid consumption is high, and the failing kidney is unable to release it in the form of urine. Aditya would have to watch his water and food consumption closely.

Aditya managed his diet as well as possible. He was pulled up on many occasions for weight gain. He tried his best not to consume more water than was permitted. But his water consumption had been very high, right from childhood.

Days of extra weight gain caused a lot of discomfort, as more water had to be drained out, leading to intense cramps. He needed someone to rub his legs so that the circulation was restored. I was at work and could not be with him at the kidney centre, so he managed on his own, suffering all kinds of discomfort without a murmur.

The hospital required the patient to be accompanied by someone, preferably a family member, during the time spent in the centre. The patient might need some assistance if he experienced cramps or nausea. My sister spent a few afternoons, but this was not possible on a long-term basis. Aditya arranged with a few friends to spend time with him at the dialysis centre, during which time they would discuss theories in physics and mathematics.

The other patients at the kidney centre were much older. Their suffering was more intense because of their age, constitution, and family responsibilities. Some were diabetic, with even greater diet restrictions, making it difficult for them to be cheerful with their lowered energy levels.

Reflections

I never heard Aditya complain that I did not give him more attention. I think he realised how much his health meant to me.

I did go to the hospital on some odd afternoon, when I could take off from work. The few times I was there, I would sit holding his arm and tears would roll down my cheeks, unintended.

I cried not only because he was my child, and he suffered. I cried because he never complained. I watched him helplessly as he bore his pain patiently. My limited participation in his treatment hurt me terribly.

That was the trade-off—either be a good mother, nursing him through the dialysis, or play it safe, with energy and time so that the transplant could happen without a hiccup. I had made a very conscious decision. It was important to preserve all my energy and be fit and ready for the transplant surgery.

As I look back, I understand the true value of such experiences. It was during those lonely and difficult times that Aditya learnt to hold the reins of his life with complete control. Realising the importance of becoming independent, he found ways to take care of his health. In doing this, he emerged as a person with a very positive outlook; he could set his objectives and list his priorities. He grew to be a determined young man, ready to fight his illness.

Paving the Way for the Transplant

February to April 1999

Sometime in February 1999, I made a special visit to Dr Gandhi. My oncologist had cleared me as fit, after I had completed both chemotherapy and radiation. Tests were done to check whether there were any active cells. Since the doctor was satisfied with my health, it was now time to offer my kidney to Aditya.

Dr Gandhi was still not comfortable. He appreciated my willingness to donate the organ, but he did not consider it advisable. He explained that even a single cancerous cell could be devastating and could spread like wildfire in a post-transplant situation, when immunity would be compromised and suppressed.

I persuaded him to have me fully tested. The transplant surgery could be contemplated if there was no threat of harm to Aditya's health. Aditya would soon be on his long summer vacation, so it would an ideal time for surgery, rest and recovery.

After repeated requests, Dr Gandhi finally relented.

He first gave me a note ordering some preliminary tests to ascertain the condition of my kidney. The tests were to check the blood group and RH factor and also included a chest X-ray, an ultrasonography of the abdomen and pelvis, an electrocardiogram, a complete blood count (CBC), and a test of blood urea nitrogen (BUN).

I was happy that we could start the process of evaluation. The tests were done at BCH, making it easy to collect reports and meet the doctor with the results. The doctor would give a cursory glance at the reports and hand me another slip for the next round of tests. The tests required were a urine sensitivity analysis and CA-153 test (Cancer Antigen 153).

"

This became a routine for the next three weeks. I would promptly show up at the kidney centre, hoping that the evaluation was completed, only to be asked for more investigations. Dr Gandhi continued to disappoint me, never telling me if the tests were favourable and whether there was reason to feel encouraged so that I might let out a sigh of relief.

Among other tests, there were a urine culture and colony count, an HIV/Australia antigen test, an antimicrobial susceptibility test, a creatinine clearance test, a liver function test, a renal profile, a renal angiography, a bone scan, an X-ray for intravenous urography and plain abdomen, and a crossmatching of donor cells with recipient serum.

By the time we finished all these and other routine tests, we were in the last week of March 1999.

As a parent it was important for me to move heaven and earth to make the kidney transplant possible. This seemed to be the single purpose in my life. I wanted to be instrumental in bringing relief to my son, affording him the chance to lead a normal life.

The medical fraternity is under oath to follow ethical practices. My family appreciated and respected that their professional reputation could be at stake by my stubborn desire to donate my kidney after my passage through cancer. But we had little option. My sister, sister-in-law, and nephews had tested, but there was no match of blood group.

Persistence helped in my breaking ground with the nephrologists, whose hesitation was well placed. I give full credit to them for checking my test reports microscopically in order to be hundred per cent confident that my past condition would not compromise my son's health.

Finally, one evening, Dr Gandhi broached the subject. He wanted us to choose the surgeon to be engaged for the surgery.

The family had already decided that we would engage the renowned urologist Dr Fardoon Sonawala. Breach Candy Hospital was well suited for a sensitive surgery requiring high levels of hygiene and nursing care. We therefore got straight into details on what the surgery would entail.

Dr Gandhi informed us of some formalities to be completed before the transplant. The Transplantation of Human Organs Act, 1994, had set up an authorisation committee responsible for approving organ donors. They approved only genuine cases. Donors were expected to be willing individuals over eighteen years of age whose blood relation could be established as a mother, father, brother, or sister of the recipient. In some cases, approval was granted to unrelated donors if there was sufficient evidence that no financial exchange was involved. Documentary evidence, affidavits to establish relationship, and a written statement that there would be no financial exchange were needed for the authorisation committee to grant approval for the transplant.

The proposal for transplant originates from the hospital, signed by the doctor recommending the transplant. The first-level screening was, therefore, at the hospital.

We met Dr Sonawala. He examined Aditya and asked routine questions about his medical history. He told us he would be adopting the traditional method of open nephrectomy. This method involves making a six- to ten- inch incision on the donor's abdomen, cutting through layers of muscle. Then the surgeon would cut and clamp the ureter and the blood vessels that connect the kidney with the bladder. After the kidney is removed, the incision is sutured. This surgical procedure would take about three hours.

Laparoscopic nephrectomy, acknowledged worldwide as superior, since it is a minimally invasive surgery, with quicker recovery time for the donor, is the more recent technique. The instruments used are long, narrow rods to view, cut and remove the kidney. It takes longer, however, than an open nephrectomy.

Since this technique was only recently introduced in India, open nephrectomy was the best option in our case. As Dr Sonawala was travelling out of the country, the only date suitable to him was 8 April 1999. With great difficulty, we managed to complete the legal formalities in time to meet the surgery's schedule.

For the post-operative care, we made several adjustments at home.

Of the three bedroom spaces, the room that was farthest from the front door, which happened to be the room Aditya shared with Dhananjay, was allotted for the post-surgery stay. The room had an attached bath and toilet facility.

The room was air conditioned, with a television and music player for entertainment, while, for communication, a telephone line and a desktop computer with Internet connection were arranged so Aditya could be actively connected to the outside world.

The bedroom door was replaced by a wooden door with a glass panel. This helped us keep track of his well-being and attend to him when he summoned us. We needed to be alert to how he was progressing.

To maintain a dust-free atmosphere, the bedroom windows were kept closed at all times. Rugs from his room and the drawing room carpet were moved into our garage so that we could clean the floors every day with disinfectants. Any chance of bacteria from carpets was to be avoided. This would provide a safe and clean environment, which is necessary for the success of an organ transplant.

Only minimum clothing was kept in the room and the cupboard. The curtains, bed sheets, and pillowcases were dry-cleaned, and Aditya's day-to-day clothes were newly sewn—free-flowing dishdasha (Arabian robes) that would not rub against the surgical stitches around his abdomen, allowing them to heal properly.

We even changed our household servants, bringing in a few efficient, clean helpers who were good at details, so that they could keep the house very clean. All this was done to ward off any lingering chance of infections.

The above arrangements were not really the standard required. Your doctor and the social worker will advise the best arrangements in your case.

With so much work done, we were ready to proceed with the surgery.

The Transplant Surgery

8 April 1999

It seems it was just yesterday.

The dark-blue overnight bag was packed and ready. It had both our medical files, personal-care items, and some clothes. These were tense moments, as one feels just before an examination.

My sister Kausalya had arrived from Madurai, offering full support and assistance. She accompanied us to the hospital on 7 April. Just as we squeezed ourselves into the car, I remembered that I had to visit the Siddhivinayak (Lord Ganesha's) temple before being hospitalised.

I prayed with deep faith, and so did Aditya. His face was serene, though one could see lines of anxiety around the corners of his small mouth.

The car entered the familiar, heavy iron gates of the Breach Candy Hospital. *That will be our home for the next few weeks,* I mused.

While we were being registered, Aditya took the flight of stairs to the first floor for a last dialysis before the surgery. The day dawned as bright and sunny as any summer morning.

I was ready for the surgery when early visitors walked in. My sisters and friends came to wish me, some with smiles lighting their faces, others wearing worried looks.

Cards and bouquets came in great numbers, and someone smeared vibuthi (religious ash) on my forehead.

There was constant news travelling between the rooms. I got minute-by-minute accounts of how Aditya was faring. He was cheerful and was waiting with bated breath, excited about the day's events. We had nearly twenty-five visitors— family members and close friends, as well as some acquaintances from the kidney centre. Everyone was there to cheer Aditya.

As the time for surgery approached, Aditya's excitement grew. He rushed into my room, holding the gown behind him to cover any exposure while dragging the intravenous (IV) stand. He was all smiles as he gushed that he just wanted to see me before the surgery.

In time, the atmosphere changed. The resident doctor injected Aditya with a sedative and moved to my room to do the same to me.

As we entered the plush, golden doors of the operation theatre, with the hospital's most modern facilities, we had a moment to ourselves; our eyes met to convey our wishes. Aditya smiled at me, and I smiled back.

That wonderful, silent moment spoke volumes.

In a few minutes the scene changed, and the moment for emotional exchanges was past. We were wheeled into two different chambers within the operation theatre. I was moved to a table that was in the centre of the room. The effects of the local anaesthesia had started kicking in. Through the haziness, I saw white curtains drawn to form a wall around me.

Then I found several human faces looking down at me. The anaesthetist smiled and introduced herself. I was aware of watching her working by my side. I closed my eyes, simply saying silently, 'All should be well.'

The next thing I recall was a dark alley. With my eyes barely open, I sensed an urgency to puke and felt uncomfortable. I was trying to wake myself. I wanted to eat.

That was the night before.

At daybreak, I was woken up by the nurse with a hot pot for steam inhalation. She did the routine blood pressure and pulse checks and also checked my temperature. The operation had lasted a little over three hours. As I regained complete consciousness, I enquired about Aditya. I was told that he had regained consciousness the previous night. I had taken much longer.

Dr Gandhi strolled in sometime later.

After a bright 'Good morning' and checking on how I was feeling, he told me that Aditya was better. He was chirpy and had read out a card that was sent by a friend. He liked the message and had asked him for a copy.

Suddenly he asked me whether there was a family history of epilepsy. Aditya had had a bout of seizures the previous night. It was surprising, as there was no such family history. Tests such as electrophysiology, a radioisotope renogram, and a CT scan of the head, checking for the existence of any lytic lesions, were conducted to find a cause for the epileptic seizures. I have a vague memory that they stopped administering Azoran, which has a tendency to bring out this reaction.

Though it was normal for a post-transplant patient to be kept in an isolated room where he received special care, with strict measures regarding hygiene, Aditya had to be shifted to the ICU for his condition to be monitored. In the ICU, visitors were permitted.

The evening was peak time for visitors. Many ladies and children from our apartment complex arrived. There was noise and chatter all around. I felt I was no longer within the confines of a hospital.

Everyone was excited about the surgery. In spite of so many organ transplants happening the world over, one is always happy to relate personal experiences. They made me feel great that I had made this organ donation. I had given another life to Aditya. I reminded them that any parent would have done this to give their child a chance to live a normal life. But they were so occupied with their chatter that my comment went unheard.

That the transplant was reasonably successful was evident from how Aditya managed an active and productive life for a few years with the transplanted kidney.

If you, reader, are placed in a similar circumstance and want to be an organ donor like me, you are seriously advised to check with your conscience and go ahead with what you believe is right.

Keen interest in donating an organ must combine with full consideration that the patient's welfare is not compromised. The donation of an organ should be a safe experience for both the donor and the recipient.

Towards this end, seek your doctor's advice and persuade him to assist you in your mission. Ensure that all tests are done and that everything is verified to full satisfaction. In case of doubt, please get a second opinion. Remember, safety is of utmost importance for both the patient and you.

After the organ donation, my health was not compromised. The joy of knowing that I had given my son some years of happiness swelled my heart with a pride of achievement. I will never experience such a feeling ever again.

Reflections

Despite five decades of successful organ transplants, this surgery continues to evoke curiosity and awe among all sectors of society. The enormity of an organ transplant is felt when suddenly the recipient's life changes and he begins to enjoy normal life. So when a transplant presents itself, people generally find reason to marvel at God's creation. This will be a hot topic for the next few days as they excitedly share their first-hand information. This experience will be a reference point for future cases of organ transplant.

The human mind has remarkable capacity to observe and store such special incidents in life for recall at an appropriate time.

I realised that all this ado was a silent tribute to God, through whom such miracles are possible.

Dedicated doctors, researchers, and medical professionals have contributed to finding remarkable solutions for many serious health problems. If detected early, there is a good chance for a cure for many kinds of cancer; restricting the spread of HIV is possible with some treatments.

Constant search is on for better, more advanced solutions like finding ways of reducing complications, giving a transplant a longer life, lowering the incidence of side effects due to prolonged medication. Experiments are tirelessly conducted to find the conclusive results of theories. It takes people with rare talent and a persuasive approach to make breakthroughs in medical research.

God has blessed them. He also provides them fresh challenges in the form of a new virus or infection that we hear and read about every other day. So there are opportunities for researchers to continuously break down the barriers and overcome their own limitations as they reach a higher level of competency.

The human body is created so magnificently that partial cure or recovery is possible. That one kidney is sufficient, and the second one in the human body a provision for mechanical failures shows excellence in design capabilities. God has engineered the human body remarkably well.

The machinery is complex, with unique power motors, intricate and well tuned, with smooth and silent functioning. He has given us vocal cords, with different volumes and amplifiers, and taste buds to enjoy different kinds of food— sweet, sour, bitter and pungent and combinations of these tastes; the ability to see the wonders of the earth and an imaginative mind that can see beyond reality.

He has connected every part of the body with cords, so that none is isolated, a liquid to keep the body running smoothly, some tools to help us move things and ourselves. He did not forget to make a strong pumphouse, to see that the fluid moves.

He wants us to take ample care of this fantastic body that he effortlessly built. Some physical problems are hereditary, but some are due to negligence/ignorance.

With the rural population, the reason for losing lives could be the unavailability of basic medical facilities (let alone the advanced medical attention needed for an organ transplant), financial deprivation, and ignorance that allows the populace little sense of reality in matters of life and death. With the media playing a role in communicating social messages, there is increasing awareness of the need for vaccination, family planning, testing for HIV and eye/ blood donations. TV campaigns are now being aired to promote kidney and other organ donations.

In larger towns and cities, there are three kinds of people. A small percentage of human beings worry without reason about their health and well-being. Some of them overdo it to the extreme and cannot see beyond themselves.

Another minuscule percentage of people worry rightly. They have knowledge, and they understand their health problem. They work towards attending to the problem in good time.

A larger population is too busy/preoccupied or simply careless. Most of us move about, oblivious of changes in our bodies, since we are completely involved in matters of everyday life such as earning a livelihood and managing the stress of an urban lifestyle. Knowledge surfaces only when we encounter a health problem. We simply live our lives as each day unfolds. Yet we are constantly worried about our future.

The human machinery is so complicated and fragile that it needs to be handled with care. Given that medicine has advanced and solutions are available, we need to acknowledge that attention is required, seek medical help and ensure that efforts are made to recover from that particular disease.

Aditya's Recovery

23 April 1999

Within a few days, Aditya was shifted back to his isolation chamber. He was on IV fluids, so he was confined to bed. There was a nurse on twenty-four-hour attendance to monitor vital signs, including measuring the urine output. Her duty also extended to giving him medication at fixed times and maintaining a record of changes in medicine, dosage, and so on. Prednisone, Imuran (azathioprine) and Neoral Sandimum (cyclosporine) were the primary medicines prescribed for safeguarding the kidney. Aditya was also to take other medicines like amlodipine, Zinetac, and Minipress at specified times.

The first day was a fluid diet, but gradually Aditya's diet improved and became near normal. He was given nutritious and light meals, with low salt and fat—vegetables normally cooked, and small portions of fruits. Soon he was able to eat regular food.

He was picking up health, and it appeared that the transplanted organ was settling in. But he suffered from extreme boredom, as visitors were directed to my room.

Post transplant, Aditya was still weak and prone to infection, as his immunity was low, so anyone entering the room was obligated to wear a mask covering the nose and mouth.

Aditya was flooded with get-well cards and messages that helped to cheer him up. Visitors brought books and magazines for his diversion. But each day, with growing energy, he wanted to take flight.

In the first fortnight after the transplant, some of the tests done before the transplant were repeated. These tests were meant to confirm normal functioning of the kidney, acceptance of the organ and assessment of whether the medication was being properly absorbed by the body. This could prompt early action if needed.

They performed an ultrasonography of the transplanted kidney. Urine cultures and sensitivity tests were conducted; clinical toxicology for cyclosporine absorption was done twice on 15 and 30 April. These tests were repeated after several months. The other tests were an electrocardiogram, chest X-ray, serum electrolytes, and blood culture, colour doppler, residual urine volume, and drainage fluid for creatinine.

The creatinine, which was at 8.8 mg/dl a day prior to transplant, was 1.3 on 21 April 1999. With the creatinine stabilising, Aditya was discharged on 23 April. He was ecstatic.

My part of the surgery involved cutting a body part, which meant substantial blood loss, making me very weak. In the comfort of home, with family showering love and attention on me, I chose to rest and recoup the lost energy. Aditya's bedroom was cordoned off. Through the glass pane on the door, we could check on him. My sister was his only visitor. She planned his meals with great enthusiasm and took care of all aspects of nutrition and hygiene.

She would check whether he had taken his medicines and record temperature and blood pressure on a chart as required by the doctor. She would hand him his meal trays and clear them after he had finished. She would spend a few minutes, chatting with him and cheering him up. The air conditioner kept the room cool round the clock, and it served to block dust. His music system and television kept him entertained. He listened to music more often than watching TV or reading so as to reduce the load on his eyes. The cleaning boy would be let into the room in the mornings. He would give Aditya's room and toilet a thorough cleaning with a generous use of disinfectants.

Aditya's clothes were given special treatment—washed separately in Dettol and ironed. Gloves were used to handle his clothes, food trays and anything else that entered his room. Aditya wore a mask whenever anyone entered his room.

We went to the hospital for regular tests and follow-ups. The blood test on 26 April showed creatinine at 1.4 mg/dl but it changed on 29 April when the report surprised us with a reading of 2.4 mg/dl. The test was repeated on the thirtieth, when it went up further, to 2.9 mg/dl.

The period for worry had begun.

Spurt of Hospitalisations

3 May to 25 June 1999

In spite of our best efforts to guard against infection, Aditya met with an episode of minor rejection on 3 May 1999, barely ten days after he had come home from the hospital.

He woke up that morning feeling slightly feverish and by one o'clock in the afternnon his temperature had shot up to 104° C. We called the doctor, who advised us to give him Crocin and bring down the temperature with ice packs. We acted as advised and managed to bring down the temperature, but it bounced back in the late afternoon.

By four o'clock, Aditya was ready to be admitted to the hospital, as we all felt that the problem would be dealt with at the hospital with prompt medical care. We were relieved to hand over care of our post-transplant patient to the hospital, with doctors monitoring his health on an hourly basis.

This did not absolve us of our worry and tension. Our apprehensions on kidney rejection made us vigilant, since this was not too far-fetched a possibility for many an organ transplant patient. This episode demanded our complete attention. Restlessness drove us down the hospital corridor to the nurses' station, where we were encouraged to wait with patience.

Patience . . . low in supply, but much needed. Agitation and fear created a complex mental state that needed conquering. We faced the chance of a setback with as much calm as we could muster, but the tension persisted.

The routine of blood tests and nurses measuring temperature and urine outputs began. The doctor informed us that it was a case of minor rejection. Treatment for anti- rejection was carried out. Aditya was administered 500 mg of methylprednisolone over two days.

The result of a blood test on 4 May showed the creatinine level as 2.1 mg. It tapered down to 1.6 mg/dl the next day and Aditya was discharged on 6 May when creatinine was at 1.4 mg/dl.

He resumed life within the sterile environment we had created at home. Our first taste of a rejection made us more watchful. It may have been overconfidence that had led us to believe that the organ had settled in properly.

Twelve days later, Aditya experienced another rise in body temperature. The doctor started him on Ceftum 500 mg, but he needed to be admitted to the hospital to be treated for viral fever. More tests became necessary, so apart from the routine CBC and BUN, the doctor wanted to repeat the ECG, blood culture, urine culture and sensitivity, colony count, Widal test (test checking for the presence of salmonella, i.e., typhoid fever), and serum electrolytes.

On 26 May the creatinine finally went down to 1.6 mg/dl. Aditya was again in the comfort of his home.

He had to be hospitalised yet again on the 1 June when the creatinine was 1.80 mg/dl. It meant heavy doses of medicine to bring it down. It came down to 1.60 mg/dl on 4 June.

But the hospital corridors beckoned us yet again on 7 June.

A renal angiography was performed. The test showed a renal artery stenosis (RAS), which could have been the reason for Aditya's unstable health.

Renal artery stenosis is the narrowing of the lining of the main artery that supplies blood to the kidney. Hypertension occurs if the stenosis results in at least seventy per cent narrowing of the renal artery. This is a secondary form of hypertension that develops as a result of another medical problem. Due to stenosis, the kidney suffers from decreased blood flow and often shrinks in size.

The doctors, including the surgeon, discussed the option of doing an angioplasty and placing a stent so that the blood flow would be uninterrupted. The general view, however, was to wait and watch before jumping in headlong to do the procedure.

Further tests—ultrasonography and bone scan—were done. With that, we returned home and had to live with the knowledge that there was an arterial stenosis and hope that it would settle down without another surgery.

As an added precaution, a renal biopsy was carried out. It was already the end of July. The persistent fevers tired

Aditya. We wondered when things would settle down and he could begin to live normally.

He had secured admission into St Xavier's College for Arts and Science for a bachelor's degree in the science stream. College had started, but Aditya was on a leave of absence.

The fever came back again.

Some more tests were done. The doctor advised an additional test to determine whether he had been infected with malaria. The test showed negative results, so he continued taking his other medications.

The period from May to August 1999, was one filled with agony and uncertainty. My sister went back home in mid-May. I had a handful of helpers who handled work in the kitchen and around the house.

I was always alone, wearing out my shoes in the passages of the hospital, sometimes on the third floor and, at other times, on the fourth floor. Srini was busy at work and Dhananjay in college, as there was no apparent reason for them to take leave. After all, it made little difference, since it was the doctors and nurses who would make recovery possible.

This period of hospitalisation was filled with anxiety. In spite of the best nursing facilities, each time Aditya was uneasy, I feared the worst. Persistent follow-up with the nurses, without exhibiting inner turmoil, smiling and getting their cooperation, was the only way to get their attention. They had other patients who were probably in more need of attention. There were moments when they saw through the charade, but that only meant a change in strategy.

The visits to the hospital helped Aditya regain his health and energy. In a quiet moment, I think he drew on his inner strength and took charge of his health. He began life with his new kidney.

Aditya's health cruised along.

Life Stabilised

I cannot put down a time or date or even a month when things changed, as far as Aditya was concerned. We were too preoccupied with attending to him, constantly on edge about his health. We were perpetually on guard against any sneeze, cold, cough and fever, so we were unaware of any change. We lived under a cloud of doubt of our capability, fearful of being 'caught napping', as it would mean very serious trouble. We lived each day as it unfolded.

We never quite knew when our sail was set in the direction of the wind, and we sailed comfortably into the deep sea of life. We were suddenly in very calm waters and, without a doubt, were enjoying the cool comfort of peace.

Aditya steadily gained stability in health. Since our first meeting with Dr Gandhi, Aditya had been made accountable for taking medicines as prescribed. There was direct dialogue between the doctor and patient on medications and their applications, so Aditya became responsible and managed them independently. The doctor found him fit to start college. His college bag had the medicine stock so that he was never stranded. The green face mask formed part of his dressing style. He wore it to college without batting an eyelid.

He soon got busy with his undergraduate curriculum. I started work as a full-time employee. My company management had shown extreme cooperation during this phase of our life.

Life now moved on.

It appeared we were strong and could control the force of the wind. Periodic medical tests and doctors' visits, along with college and its exams, were part of life's routine.

It needed some courage to ask Aditya how he felt. 'So . . . Aditya, how are you?'

'It's so nice to be back to doing something. College is good. I have made new friends. Everyone is busy with work. They stop to ask about my mask. When I talk about my transplant, they look surprised. They wonder how I seem so unaffected.'

Then, with some emotion and earnestness, he said, 'Amma, you know what? I am very happy to be able to pass urine properly. This is the first time. All this time . . . I never felt so good when I passed urine.'

It was poignant, unbelievable, and unimaginable. Nobody made such assessments of a kidney function, but here was Aditya actually complimenting it. He was feeling good, doing a normal everyday activity which we all take for granted. His statement made me realise how much relief his new kidney had given him. I also wondered how many times as a kid he had experienced discomfort. It's sad that I did not know anything about those uncomfortable moments.

Aditya contemplated deeply how to improve his life and career. In college he made some good friends with girls and boys who were intellectually compatible and had similar interests. Though the students were curious about the mask they soon appreciated his predicament and boosted his ego with their support.

The mask was on for only a few months, as Aditya believed he should become constitutionally strong and should be able to withstand every infection by increasing his immunity. He travelled to college in a car and avoided crowded buses and theatres. As we lived in the cleaner environment of Pedder Road, he was safer. So we accepted this theory. (But between you and me, my heart would come to a standstill at the slightest change in his health. My mind was loaded with unexplainable worry.)

As he grew healthier, Aditya started actively planning his life and career. He developed a close relationship with his professors and took their advice on courses he should pursue. They guided him, took interest in his work and gave him opportunities to present case studies. He was working fast towards his goals. All career plans revolved round his health condition. Though Aditya would never permit his health to deter his progress or set the framework for his work, he made choices that would encompass all aspects without holding him back. He was not bound by any limitations on what he could achieve.

With great grit and determination, he steered his life from the dullness that had engulfed him since November 1996. The transplant brought a new meaning to his life. He braved the toughest period with a smile brightening his face. Now his happiness knew no bounds. He wanted to live every moment to its fullest. He made tough decisions about his career without once wondering how he would manage.

Of the four of us, he was the strongest. His 'never-give- up spirit' became the guiding light for the rest of us. Unknowingly, we drew our inspiration of life from him.

He brought so much cheer into our lives that our eyes became dry as though for eternity. He never stood back, reflecting on what he had passed through, but marched ahead with full command over his life. He was very passionate about life and wanted to live it to the fullest.

He pursued physics and mathematics. Theories of relativity, quantum mechanics, and nanotechnology featured in his discussions. He spoke of these topics with great zeal. I would hear it all and not understand a word. As an emotional mother, my mind would zoom around, wondering, hoping and praying that his dreams should materialise.

Every opportunity to travel out of Mumbai to participate in seminars or summer research would engage his interest. Even if there were limited seats, he somehow managed to secure a placement. It did not bother him that he had a bag full of medicines to tow along.

As for us, we agitated and made great efforts to tie him down to a less rigorous lifestyle, keeping his health as our main focus. He showed us the importance of giving him his freedom to grow without any boundaries. On his own, he had set down his daily diet regime, sometimes saltless and sometimes treating himself to something that he loved.

All he wanted was to see the world, enjoy meeting new people, making friends, expanding his career opportunities and his horizon of visualisation.

The family supported him, as we realised that there was no apparent reason to curb his growth. He was extremely responsible, and it was important for him to handle his life and career independently. The family stood by, respecting his sentiments.

During that time, Dr Stephen Hawking toured India and came to Mumbai. Aditya managed to get a free pass to attend his lecture on the theory that black holes remit radiation, at the Homi Bhabha Auditorium, and he was thrilled about it. He took great inspiration from Hawking, who managed so well in spite of the motor neuron disease that had left him almost completely paralysed.

Aditya developed an interest in music. He wanted to learn to play the guitar. He was a self-learner, so he downloaded music notes from the Internet and started strumming. His guitar would be all over the house. Late at night after the household became silent, he would open doors to the world of music as he enjoyed playing his guitar in the silence of the night.

Around this time, Dhananjay conveyed his decision to seek admission for a master's in electrical engineering in Los Angeles's University of Southern California (USC). Later, he graduated from this university and then headed for a job in the Silicon Valley.

In the meantime, Aditya finished his three-year course of undergraduate study and fared very well. This helped him in obtaining admission to the Indian Institute of Technology in Powai and Rourkee. He selected the Institute at Powai for his choice of subjects. He lived in the hostel and ate meals there. He was careful to eat only hot meals so that the hygiene factor was taken care of.

In 2004, he finished his master's and chose to do a PhD. He had offers from the Tata Institute of Fundamental Research (TIFR), Satyen Bose Institute, and several American universities. He chose the University of Southern California in Los Angeles.

The doctor was happy with the progress of his health. The creatinine bordered around 1.6 mg/dl, and Aditya's health was steady enough for him to take another plunge. On 23 July 2004, he left for the United States. He lived with a group of Indian friends. He cooked meals at home. Eating out was restricted to Subway restaurants and other establishments that served fresh food. He was careful about the salt content and purchased groceries after studying the labels for nutritional facts.

This period of life continued to be a high, as far as Aditya's career was concerned. He progressed well in his doctoral studies. He managed to do wonderfully, published papers within a year, represented and participated on behalf of USC at various seminars and conferences in New York, Boston, Denver, Houston, among several other places.

He initiated treks with his graduate students or stayed in overnight camps. During this phase he developed an interest in photography and, with an SLR and a tripod, he went capturing pictures of interest.

He worked hard, as if attempting to excel at everything he did. His cooking capabilities were already established when he was still in school, and now he discussed food, read recipe books with me, cooked restaurant-style paneer butter-masala, and pottered around the kitchen, almost wanting to take it over from me.

Aditya was living his dream life and enjoying every bit of it.

The Debacle

It was December 2005 and winter had set in. It was celebration time the world over. Aditya called. He had this frightful cold. None of the home remedies and treatments of hot-water inhalation had helped. Not even the normal analgesics recommended for kidney patients had given him relief.

He complained of headaches, fever and cold and, above all, general weakness. I kept pleading with him to get some medical help. A few days later, he moved into Dhananjay's apartment in Mountain View, a suburb of San Francisco.

His health continued to deteriorate, but he persisted with his smiling assurances that all was well. Dhananjay was cooking him hot meals while he rested.

New Year dawned. My husband had, in the meantime, taken up a job in Dubai. I had quit my job and had planned to move to Dubai to live with him.

On 3 January, the telephone rang. The call was from Dhananjay.

'Amma . . . there's some news. Aditya is not well and we have hospitalised him.'

'But what happened?'

'He was breathless, so we did a blood test at the OPD. They found his creatinine as high as 20 mg/dl, and potassium was at 11 mg. He is at Stanford Hospital and Clinics in the ER. With enemas the potassium has been brought down.'

I neither talked nor did I think. I just listened.

Dhananjay comforted me the best he could and promised to keep me updated.

I knew I had to make a trip to the United States. The process of getting a visa and arranging my travel took a couple of days. The calls and updates came, reassuring me. But I was still disturbed by thoughts revolving around Aditya. I wanted to be there by his bedside.

In the meantime, the hospital had put him on dialysis to reduce the creatinine. Palo Alto's Stanford Hospital gave him three doses of Solumedrol (methylprednisolone) 500 mg through an IV. Aditya was on a three-hour dialysis schedule, three times a week.

I reached the hospital in a daze. I believed naively that my being there would do the miracle.

The biopsy report showed acute rejection, and there were indications of humoral rejection. I shared these findings with Dr Gandhi, who concurred with the treatments offered and continued to offer support long-distance.

After receiving emergency treatment, Aditya was discharged from the hospital. A few more dialysis sessions were scheduled.

Being born in a different era, all Aditya could think of was showing me around San Francisco. Still not recovered from jet lag and in a state of shock, I went on the sightseeing trips without giving a thought to whether it was appropriate. Any other mother would have found solace in prayers or in seeking more information of her child's health condition.

Dhananjay took leave from work and drove us to Los Angeles. We met Dr Mohammed Akmal, who was Aditya's designated nephrologist at the University of Southern California's hospital. The doctor was briefed on what had happened during the Christmas holidays. The attending doctors from Stanford Hospital had sent all the reports to Dr Akmal, which gave him advance notice of Aditya's kidney rejection.

All tests, including the biopsy, were repeated at the USC Hospital. The full impact of the rejection came out in the open. The doctor promised to give treatment for reviving the functions. During his ten days' stay at the hospital, Aditya was given three doses of Prednisolone, an anti- rejection drug, through IV. This biopsy too showed two different rejections—humoral rejection, which is a chronic condition, and also an acute rejection.

Realising that the body was resisting cyclosporine, the doctor changed the immunosuppressant medication to Prograf. Dr Akmal held a conference with his team of doctors and decided on the next line of treatment. They started Aditya on thymoglobulin (three IVs), followed by plasmapheresis (removing the plasma from his blood and infusing fresh plasma and albumin) to arrest further damage to the kidney by the antibodies in the plasma which were attacking the transplanted kidney. The treatment was completed with an intravenous immunoglobulin (IVIG).

The team of doctors at USC acted quickly and took an aggressive approach to arrest further damage. Clearly all measures were taken to recover the kidney. The kidney function was expected to be revived and last for a few years, if the treatment succeeded.

The mother in me kept wishing, 'If we got the kidney working for a few years, we would have time to plan his second transplant.'

We waited with patience, hoping there would be signs of recovery. Everyone in the family was very concerned. We contacted some distant relatives based in the United States and their friends in the medical community. Nothing much could be done, however, as any action taken would be by the attending doctors. Clearly, the case was studied from all angles by the USC team.

All we could do was to wait for results.

In the meantime, Aditya continued the thrice-a-week dialysis schedule at a satellite unit of DaVita, which in Spanish means 'one who gives life'.

DaVita's centre at USC had over forty dialysis units, with three schedules a day, so that about 240 patients were dialysed in a week. DaVita's size of operations was not the same across all cities, as some centres had fewer units. They operated in more than forty-three states in the United States, with over 1,400 outpatient dialysis facilities. They had a facility for organising vacation dialysis at any of these centres.

This comforted Aditya, since he could continue to travel within the United States.

Dr Akmal attended on him and monitored him closely, to be sure he settled well. A doctor has to not only act as a physician but also handle the psychological aspects of the patient's well-being.

Aditya had accepted the setback cheerfully. That is the most wonderful thing about him. I thank God for giving him this quality.

Days passed and grew into weeks of waiting. When we questioned, the doctors continued to encourage us to wait. Aditya would analyse the reports and tell me that the possibility of recovery was very dim. It seemed that I was the only one hoping that his kidneys would restart.

Reflections

Life is not only a journey of success and happiness. The journey needs to be spiked with excitement, moments of worry, sorrow and difficulties in order for us to learn and enjoy life in its completeness. Change, they say, is constant. Six and a half years was a long time to live happily. This period had made us complacent, lethargic. Our grip had loosened. It had been difficult to retain a hold on the sail.

The winds had grown stronger.

We struggled and thumped and did everything possible to pull back the sail, but it refused to be set in the direction of the wind. We tried to get help from knowledgeable people. They tried but shook their heads in regret. It was impossible to get the ship sailing as we desired.

All efforts combined could not produce the desired magic, because the sea was too violent. The sail could not be held back by mere human hands. It needed something more powerful to curb it.

The dice was cast. It was a loss. It was time to move on! I felt very, very sad that Aditya lost his kidney. It worried me endlessly, since he would now pass through a tough phase, handling dialysis on his own; all alone, all by himself, with only his friends to support him. I couldn't be with him for long to manage his diet and health.

He had to manage his meals, attend school, do his research, drive to DaVita for his dialysis and manage his Teaching Assistantship (TA). It was a tight schedule. I spent four months helping him settle into this lifestyle. My emotions and over-protective attitude at the second phase of dialysis were holding back his progress on research. I needed him on his front foot always.

This was yet another important experience in life. To handle and overcome the emotional issues even while progressing into the next stage in life.

Aditya was his usual self, not cringing. He assumed his role of a caretaker, while I watched in pained silence, praying for his well-being. The task of finding a kidney was now difficult. Where would we find one? We were more worried now as fewer solutions emerged.

Reflections

Life is a great mystery. The more we try to solve it, the more we get involved. The situation gets complicated, as we want immediate results.

There is no magic formula for achieving our dreams. Everything needs time and patience till we can finally hit the button of success. Until that time, we must simply permit life to take its course.

In that alone will there be peace.

Sense and Sensibility

Sense

he day before I left Los Angeles, Dhananjay, Aditya and I spent the afternoon checking out the water at Venice Beach. We were standing with feet soaked in the slightly cold water, when Aditya threw his arm across my shoulders. Dhananjay came across and held me at the waist.

In a quiet voice, Aditya looked upward and with his fingers he drew on the blue sky the course of life after transplant.

He said, 'Three years at St Xavier's College—hectic, with papers in math; working closely with Prof Patwardhan and then . . . two years at the Indian Institute of Technology . . . interesting period . . . growth and development . . . substantial work done . . . I also had unlimited fun . . . this was somehow a very satisfying period in life . . . there was the summer school at Indian Institute of Science . . . the paper handled from back home . . . Applying to various universities for the doctorate in India and abroad . . . Satyen Bose's offer . . . first one, really . . . Choosing between the University of Southern California, LA, and Mumbai's Tata Institute of Fundamental Research—both good . . . was keen on TIFR, too . . . but settled with USC and Dr Stephan Haas . . . extensive work with him . . . the large group of IITans was a major plus . . . And a working kidney for over a year and half in the US, allowing a gradual build-up in terms of achievements . . . So, Amma, in these six and a half years I have achieved so much!'

Dhananjay and I looked at each other silently, eyes gradually filling with knowing wonder. It was indeed a good recount of the events in his life, so packed, so much accomplished, and Aditya's spirit still intact after the misfortune of losing a kidney!

He had shown me that he had understood the value of his life, and felt that within a short time what he had achieved was beyond his expectations. I was dumbstruck by the newfound realisation that there was so much reason for gratitude. I felt like a fool for worrying endlessly about my son.

We stood looking at the distant horizon beyond the wide expanse of blue sea, the sky streaked with shades of orange, red and yellow as the sun shied away, ready to bid me good-bye.

This image imprinted itself in my mind's eye as one depicting the shades of life: Hope—seeing the wonderful waves soaring high as if wanting to touch the soft, white feathers of the seagulls; Anger—knowing that life was filled with trials and need for enormous energy to overcome them; Love of Life—deep sorrows caused by failures, happiness drawn from acceptance, and paying homage to the spirit of life.

Success is learning to accept life with all its limitations and live cheerfully.

I went back to Dubai feeling much lighter.

Sensibilities

I walked with great difficulty through the Arabian Desert, as the warm sand slipped into my shoes now and then. It did not matter too much. My thoughts were elsewhere, far away, with Aditya and Dhananjay. At a distance, I could see Srini trudging along with equal indifference.

My heart still had a deep passion for life, understanding, and a tinge of wonder. There was love and hurt. But I had resigned silently, accepting the events as charted by the universe. All our efforts were insufficient to change the course of the wind or reduce the intensity of the sun's heat or control the flow of water. There was no controlled anger. There was some peace and calm.

At the moment, nothing could be done but pray.

There was a spark of hope; the cinders were still aflame in my eyes. We could manage to live the next few years of our lives with that flame of hope. Over time the hollowness in life would be filled by joy and happiness. Wise men say, time is a great healer.

There was no sense of urgency to do anything. We sat on the warm, desert sand quiet, rested.

As night fell upon us, the sky was as dark as could be, dotted with small specks of silvery stars. From across the sky the moon shone, lighting up the night sky.

It was a very beautiful scene, there in the desert sands with the whole sky and universe all to us.

My thoughts went back to the subject, our own small world and our problems. I thought of my sons.

It was several—no, many—hours later that I was broken out of my reverie. Srini pointed to the east, where the early rays of the sun were breaking through the clouds. We watched the sunrise over a mound of desert sand. It magically transformed the sand into sparkling pieces of gold.

I smiled with the knowledge that we have to only wait for another dawn.

Someday, the sun will do wonders to our small world too.

Accepting Kidney Rejection

After my return from Los Angeles, in spite of Aditya's philosophical description of his achievements and my own feeling of lightness, my mind had lost its calm. The daily calls and e-mails did not appease me. I sought more comfort. Nagging worry about life with dialysis played in my mind. I wished I could do something to bring him relief.

The first option that I was tempted to explore was to look for unrelated donors. I visited places in India where aggressive transplants were undertaken. They even made adjustments in dosage of the immunosuppressant drugs to improve the chances for organ acceptance. This was particularly useful in cases where the tissue match was not within acceptable limits.

But when I was close to finding some links, I called Aditya to share my findings. His first reaction was what he had said before his first transplant, 'I am not interested in an unrelated donor.'

But, to my horror, after some thought, he said, 'And . . . Amma, I will not have another transplant.' He added uneasily, 'It is too much responsibility to take care of a kidney.' I thought he felt that in a sense he had let me down.

This reminded me of our conversation a few months after the rejection episode. Aditya had been watching me closely; to him, hurt was evident in my eyes. Of course he was right, but my hurt came from the suddenness of the incident that had reversed his life. It was more worry about his life ahead. I would see him leave for dialysis before daybreak on the appointed days and returning home briefly for breakfast before proceeding to university. Life would be tough for him, with so many activities packed into a day.

One day he said to me, 'Amma, I feel sorry seeing you so troubled. I should have taken better care of your kidney.'

This took me by surprise, and I immediately retaliated, 'That kidney was no longer mine. So I have no hard feelings, you know. What really bothers me is that dialysis will drain you of energy.' I added endearingly, 'Chico, I worry about you—nothing more.'

His face lit up with relief as he said, 'Thank God. I was feeling irresponsible.'

After breaking our reserve months ago, this conversation now was leading us to another deadlock. I pursued a new line of thought, saying, 'Sometimes things do go wrong, you know, but maybe next time it will be better.' I tried consoling him while trying to understand the underlying meaning of those words.

As if reading my thoughts, he continued, 'Kidney transplant is a huge responsibility. One has to take care of so many things—taking medicines, ensuing hygiene, etc . . . it's too much work . . . I am bored.'

Definite closure of his dialogue left little leeway for me to wriggle into his private space, to get a handle on him. I wanted to know why his attitude had changed.

I felt more distanced from him than the physical distance from Dubai to Los Angeles. What he had said was something I had never heard him express before. My heart was filled with sadness. How would I ever reach out to Aditya again? The experience seemed to have soured him in a way least expected.

Reflections

Losing a kidney brings the same emotion as losing someone close to you. One cannot mourn the loss of a kidney, but the hopelessness of the situation is immeasurable and saps your energy to the core. One cannot see the road ahead.

Unfortunately, the only question people have for the person losing his kidney is, 'How did it happen?'

Though it is in some way a show of concern, it becomes an insensitive question. Naturally, the patient plays many emotional battles within, including blaming himself. So the best thing would be to show love and understanding. After all, even if the person was responsible for the loss, he is not exactly rejoicing about that mistake. It was unintended, and the patient pays heavily for this negligence by going back into dialysis, which isn't the easiest of setbacks! The patient experiences one of the greatest losses of his life. To regain the lost position depends on the availability of another kidney. How many will be fortunate enough to get a second chance?

The person who faces a kidney failure needs 'concern' to be replaced by 'understanding' of the need for privacy. Discussions on unrelated matters or talking about how organ rejection is quite common and of other people experiencing it, is more appropriate and encouraging.

Not all patients possess a positive attitude.

Dr Susan Conley, Physician Advisor, Utilisation and Case Management, St Christopher's Hospital for Children, Philadelphia, has set up a website linking parents and families of paediatric kidney patients for interacting with problems faced by them.

In one of her early introductory notes for nephkids, I read this note which made good sense to me:

By far, the most common reason for loss of the kidney after the first year is noncompliance with the medical regimen—missing doses of medication, which I am convinced, is sometimes done without the patient even realising it is happening, or not monitoring one's health. I think that especially in the pediatric patient that frequent blood draws are the best way to keep a handle on what is happening.

And then there are teenagers, who not infrequently decide that the kidney was meant to be theirs, so stop the meds on purpose. It may seem to work for a while not to take their medications, but it eventually is trouble.

It is difficult to deal with keeping track of whether a teen takes the meds. They have to be given some autonomy, and you can't watch their every move—so how do you monitor? My best suggestion is monthly blood draws with drug levels—cyclosporine or tacrolimus (Prograf, FK) levels, I mean, and prayers that if noncompliance occurs you'll catch it soon enough. Of course the other key is good communication with your teen and frequent discussion of the importance of taking care of the kidney.

Reading this helped me breathe easy again. Knowing that this was a common youth syndrome and my son had belonged to that group, made me less alarmed. I knew that this was no time to counsel. This was the time to heal with soothing words, with love, with encouragement. With the passage of time, I knew I would be able to reach out to Aditya as a mother would to her son.

Beyond Turbulence

2006-2007

Sometime in October 200€, Aditya had shingles or Ramsay's Hunt Syndrome and was hospitalised. He had developed herpetic lesions on the right side of his tongue, lower lip, face, and the pinna of his right ear. But Aditya's infection was severe and threatened to impair his hearing. Fortunately, it was only temporarily affected.

Through this illness Aditya stayed strong, with Dr Akmal aggressively handling treatment.

We were worried, but Dhananjay wrote to us that, apart from pain in the head and his right side affected by the infection, Aditya was overall in good condition.

How he managed this illness was a wonder. He was alone in the hospital, since this was an infectious disease, and mingling with friends was not advisable. On the one hand he was fighting pain and on the other, the fear of losing his hearing. Being a mother, I could read the underlying agony and pain during the telephone calls. Every time I threatened to come to the United States, he would assure me that he was fine. I was left confused as ever. I lost my peace of mind. Neither could I go to the United States and upset the stability of his life, nor was I happy just standing by inactive. The uncertainty of his health was uppermost in my mind and left me restless.

Springing back to health, Aditya chose to avoid further discussion, and we were hopeful that all was well.

We planned a family reunion during the winter holidays of 2006. Both Aditya and Dhananjay took a holiday with us in Mumbai, where we were among family and friends. Aditya's face masked real emotions as he played the super- cool young man and even encouraged me to smile.

The next year began with inconsequential things. All we could do was wonder about Aditya's health. He filled us with happy details of how dialysis was the best of treatments. It was no big deal, and he managed well. My every concern he blew out of the window, and he talked more of things other than health.

While Aditya had supposedly settled down with haemodialysis, he investigated the possibility of doing peritoneal dialysis. It would give him some more quality- time for his research, which was getting neglected due to his preoccupation with health care.

Aditya wrote to the family explaining why he found peritoneal dialysis a better way to continue his treatment:

Peritoneal dialysis (PD) makes use of the area in the body called the peritoneum. In this region, the body has a naturally existing semi-permeable membrane which is what is made use of. A set of catheters will be installed in that area so that the dialysis solution can fill up that region and allow for removal of wastes from the peritoneum.

The advantage of PD is that you don't have to go for dialysis two or three times a day. You have to keep the dialysis solution in your body throughout the day, remove it at night, or replace it every six hours. That's a little difficult, if I'm going to be in school, but there is another option, keep the fluid in the peritoneum during the day, and at night attach yourself to an auto-exchanger. This machine automatically exchanges fluid from the peritoneum (that was filled in the night before) with a fresh solution called dialysate. By these exchanges the body gets cleaned. All you do is attach yourself to this machine and sleep. Throughout the night the cleaning happens.

The advantages of PD are that you have a more flexible lifestyle . . . you can travel without worrying about scheduling dialysis, etc. your diet is a lot less restricted . . . the problem with haemodialysis is that you build up fluids and wastes in your body over two to three days and then remove it all in like three hours   it's very drastic . . . not good for the body, in the long run   that's why you have to be on a strict diet . . . so that your body doesn't have to routinely go through drastic effects.

On the other hand, in PD   you are either continuously cleansing the body (if you decide to do exchanges throughout the day) or you will be cleaning it once a day, at night   which is definitely better than once in two to three days.

The disadvantages . . . installing the catheters in the peritoneum requires a lot of responsibility   I have to keep the catheters clean so that I don't get any infections in that area. That's a major concern.

The main reason why I want to do peritoneal is that I like to travel around . . . for instance I was selected to attend a summer school in Italy this June. Thought the summer school was tailor-made for me, very close to my research, so made me really feel that I should attend it . . . but now, I can't with haemodialysis! So that's why I say that peritoneal is a better solution for someone who wants to lead an active life.

For a person who had an abdominal surgery like a transplant, there could be some issues regarding using the peritoneal cavity for dialysis. The urologist examined Aditya to ascertain whether his peritoneal cavity could be used for dialysis.

Finally, on 7 August 2007, Aditya underwent a surgery during which a catheter was placed in the peritoneum. This was the important connection in peritoneal dialysis that would need special care. He trained extensively with the dialysis team at DaVita, who helped him settle into PD. It was an exhaustive training, covering all details.

Better Dialysis, Better Lifestyle

Aditya had chosen the Continuous Cycling Peritoneal Dialysis (CCPD) that is done through the night. He was now in total charge of his health care. He got accustomed to high levels of hygiene and cleanliness, kept records of his BP and weight, efficiently managed his medications, and improved his diet by eating high-protein, high-calorie diets. Life changed for him now, since with continuous cleaning of his blood, he was physically relieved and more comfortable, he was more relaxed about his diet, and he could have flexibility of time for working, meeting friends and enjoying life.

Aditya was feeling high. He could plan his life better and he saw reason to be happier. With all this change came a bag-load of responsibilities.

As he was dialysed at home, he became personally involved in every stage of dialysis each night. Setting up the dialysis equipment was very procedural and required great alertness, as there was a high level of precision involved at each stage. No part of the activity could be delegated.

He received six weeks of training under the direction of Sister June P. Fung, a specialised PD nurse, who demonstrated how to connect efficiently while minimising chances of infections.

Under Aditya's purview was the responsibility of ordering the dialysis supplies with sufficient stock for ten days or more, covering for any unavoidable delays in delivery. The stock needed proper storing in clean conditions, without being exposed to adverse weather conditions. The dialysis solution should be well sealed, and there should be no leakage. Supplies that are damaged must be disposed of. The fluid outputs should be checked to see if they are clear. If the fluid is hazy, the dialysis nurse should be contacted. The catheter, which was placed on the peritoneum, had an open end that came out from the abdomen. It was closed with a flexi-disconnect cap when the dialysis was over, and the catheter was not in use. Since it was fixed to an opening in the body it needed protection from dust and other foreign particles that could infect the body.

So Aditya had to follow the standard procedure for keeping the catheter and exit site dry and clean, especially after a shower. It could also be dressed with gauze. When he started the process of setting up his dialysis, special care was needed to ensure that everything related to and touched by him was kept sterile. Cleaning with hand sanitisers was the first easy step towards hygienic peritoneal dialysis. Keeping record of BP and weight were equally important. Weight gain could mean he was under-dialysed, while weight loss would indicate the need for a better diet.

It was critical for Aditya to remember to take his medicines as prescribed. Particularly in PD, he had to be aware of the monthly blood-test results for potassium, phosphorus, BUN, albumin, calcium and haemoglobin. Changes in these chemical compositions could be directly related to medicines, diet, and dialysis. He learned to understand the changes in his blood composition from the previous test results, discuss with the doctor, and see if any change in medicines or dosages was desired.

When the haemoglobin was low, the doctor would recommend Epogen injections on a weekly basis in order to stimulate red-cell production. The dosage would be determined based on haematocrit/ haemoglobin and erythropoietin (EPO) levels. Aditya needed to remove prescribed dosage from vials for self-injecting. The dosage was reduced or increased after every lab report was scrutinised. It meant preserving these medications properly and injecting only the recommended dosage on the same day of each week.

In haemodialysis, this is handled by the clinic staff. But with this responsibility, Aditya got even closer to understanding the involvement of medicines with his health and well-being.

Curtain on Reality

The year 2007 Christmas holidays saw us in San Jose with Dhananjay.

Aditya's life, revolving round peritoneal dialysis, was supposedly giving him great comfort, so we decided to enjoy the holidays with our sons.

Aditya drove down to San Jose with the car's trunk loaded with PD equipment and supplies.

We planned a two-day visit to San Francisco, where we would spend New Year's Eve. Everyone was relaxed. We watched the fireworks, spent time sending greetings to family and friends, and, while the boys partied with friends, we settled down to watching television.

Later we were awakened by a dismayed Aditya, whose cycler machine was not performing properly. The drainage was a problem.

We left next morning for Stanford Hospital and Clinics where Aditya was admitted a second time. He was found to be highly constipated and was treated accordingly. But Aditya was not satisfied. He felt it had to be something more; he had experienced unbearable pain and discomfort during dialysis, when there was a pull in the abdomen.

While in intense pain, he shocked us by disclosing how this problem had disturbed him on many a night. He would change his posture, trying to get the right angle for the catheter to draw out the fluid. Slowly it dawned on me that Aditya had not been forthcoming about the hardships he faced. In some way he hesitated or did not want to bother us. This disturbed me endlessly.

Srini and I drove with Aditya to Los Angeles and went straight to the clinic to understand the phenomena. Dr Akmal suspected that his omentum was wrapped around the catheter and scheduled an appointment with a reputed urologist. The omentum is a sheet of fat that is covered by the peritoneum. It has the tendency to protect the body from infections, and it attacks a foreign object. In this case, the catheter was the foreign object and hence its target.

Occasionally, fibrinogen clusters would diffuse into the drain fluid. Usually these clusters could be ignored. In rare cases, however, the clusters were large and blocked the passage of the draining fluid, causing insufficient drainage and some amount of pain. Aditya had found fibrinogen on several occasions. He had infused a prescribed dose of an anticoagulant called heparin in the dialysis fluid to break the formation of fibrinogen clusters. The nurses at DaVita had taught Aditya the necessary precautions for putting this infusion directly into the dialysis solution.

So we were not sure whether it was the omentum or fibrinogen.

But the drainage problems persisted, along with the pain. The scans conducted under the urologist's recommendation showed that the omentum had tightly gripped the catheter.

A minor surgery was done at the City of Angeles Medical Center involving clamping the catheter on the sides of the abdomen.

The surgery seemed to cure the problem, but now unsure about everything, I chose to stay back in Los Angeles with Aditya till things settled with his PD. Srini returned to Dubai and to work.

The omentum continued to wreak havoc, causing Aditya sleepless nights. Aditya repeated his experiment of changing his posture every now and then, hoping that the drainage would somehow improve. But the problem persisted, and the doctors suggested removing the omentum surgically.

Therefore, another surgery was scheduled at Saint Vincent Medical Center. The urologist stapled the omentum firmly at various points on the abdomen, putting an end to the problem.

In peritoneal dialysis, Aditya continued to meet with some restriction on consuming products high in potassium. Phosphorus was still restricted. With its daily dialysis exchanges in PD, waste was removed more efficiently. The prescribed diet in peritoneal dialysis was nutritious and well-balanced meals. A higher portion of foods with high biological value or good-quality proteins was essential, as amino acids from the protein were removed during the dialysis exchange.

As a vegetarian, getting the right quality protein became a huge challenge for Aditya. Beans (beans, lentils, and other legumes) were fairly high in protein value but were also high in phosphorus. Increased dosage of phosphorus binders was unable to maintain phosphorus within limits.

The binders could help only to a certain point, beyond which there needed to be restriction in consumption of foods that vegetarians relied heavily on—legumes and dairy products—which contribute to higher phosphorus. Increased dosage of binders was not recommended, since there could be side effects.

Aditya adopted a major change by experimenting with chicken and fish, which gave him good protein. Initially he found difficulty in cooking and eating non-vegetarian meals. But over time, as his lab results for albumin became greater than four (which is a desired level for building and maintaining the cells of body such as bone, skin, hair, and muscles), he accepted this change and moved on. As he had no previous experience in cooking non-vegetarian meals, he promptly attended cooking classes where he learned to clean, cut and cook meat, including the basics of marinating fish and chicken.

With this change, his fight for lowering phosphorus ended as blood-test results showed potassium and phosphorus levels were at acceptable levels. With PD he could occasionally consume small portions of potatoes, tomatoes and spinach, which were high in potassium, without major problems.

The only great issue with the PD diet was constipation. The low-fibre food consumed by kidney patients does not provide enough roughage. The fact that white flour is better than wholewheat flour is the greatest letdown in the kidney patient's diet. Living with this diet makes the patient prone to suffering from severe constipation. Constipation could even block free access for fluid drainage, leading to inadequate or poor-quality dialysis.

Treatment for constipation through medication is possible, but in very severe cases, it has to be treated in the hospital. Aditya was advised to take a stool softener or a laxative on a daily basis for smooth bowel movements.

This phase of his life was marred now and then by problems. That made Aditya sometimes wary, while I was perpetually on tenterhooks.

But he made every attempt to remain cheerful and make the best of his life. He managed trips to Yosemite Park several times with the cycler machine, supplies and all. A dolly was part of his travel entourage. It helped to convey the heavy boxes of supplies and accessories like drain bags, connectors, masks, and hand sanitisers that were essential for his dialysis. Movies, concerts, and nightlife were also possible if dialysis was properly scheduled.

By doing this he managed to enjoy his kind of good- quality life on peritoneal dialysis.

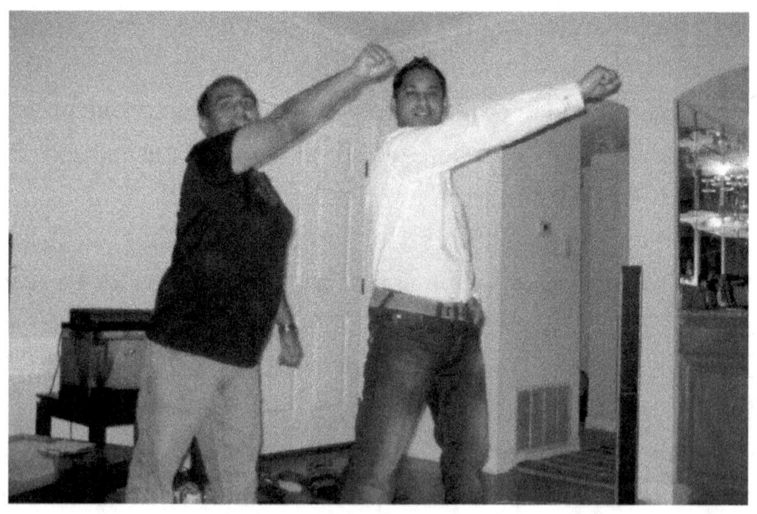

Aditya with friend Sachin on 8 August 2008 at the
release of Bollywood's *Singh is Kinng*

Life with PD

Though Aditya reiterated that life with PD was fun, he faced many problems all throughout.

The worst was yet to come.

He brought home a pet cat from the shelter. The cat was well trained, and he convinced me that his blood pressure would be under control, as pets are generally believed to help in bringing it down. To prove his statement, he produced published literature. Gamow thrilled him, and, I realised, fulfilled his need to connect with someone close—a sweetheart, maybe. The pain he had been subjected to in the past two years made him seek some close company. Even as a kid he had wanted a pet dog or cat, so now he was fulfilling his dream. He needed something to cheer him, since, even though he smiled and claimed dialysis to be very convenient, there was more to it than that. After all, for him, dialysis had also become a boring routine with the continuous monitoring of health and diet.

Though his group of friends was encouraging and very helpful, he just needed something more in the area of love. I was happy to see him cheerful, enjoying playing with Gamow. I knew it would be heartless if I were to refuse him his joy. Initially I dreaded the touch of the little one. But the beauty that she was, she charmed her way into my heart.

Keeping factors of hygiene in accordance with norms, we maintained a steady life with PD. I even helped in keeping the litter box clean so that the chance of infection was negligible. But Gamow was very spirited and mischievous and kept us on our toes. She managed to destroy many a battery charger for cell phones and laptops, as she was teething. Aditya was careful while doing dialysis, or so it seemed.

It happened in the month of May 2008 during my visit to South Bay to be with Dhananjay. One evening Aditya started vomiting. He was breathless and very unwell. He called 911. His next call was to tell me how uneasy he felt. He sounded weak. When I called back, he was not contactable. My stomach was tight with tension. The ambulance had taken him to Olympia Hospital. I had barely been with Dhananjay for two days, but Aditya's call beckoned me. So, booking the first flight out of San Jose, I made my way to the hospital.

Things needed organising. With help from Aditya's friends, I managed to take the cycler machine and supplies to the hospital for his dialysis. Blood tests were done, but the results were yet to come. Dr Akmal advised us to have Aditya transferred to the USC hospital so that he could be under his care. Olympia Hospital discharged him the next day.

At the USC hospital, Aditya's health was monitored and medications for nausea and pain were administered. Since the results of the blood tests done at Olympia Hospital were yet to be received, he was put into haemodialysis so that the peritoneum was rested.

By day two, Aditya's health had deteriorated. He puked . . . five . . . six . . . ten . . . fifteen . . . twenty . . . thirty and many more times. I was kept busy running with the bowl between bed and toilet to clean it as even the hospital nurse could not attend to one patient with such frequency.

Aditya was red in the face, the muscles on his forehead and neck stretched, showing agitation. The repeated nausea and throwing up kept him troubled and exhausted. At this stage he was off food completely. He would remain in that state till all the infection was cleared from his body. When I expressed concern, the doctor suggested inserting a nasogastric tube (NG tube).

The next morning, the tube was inserted through Aditya's nose to bring out the remnants of infection, toxicity from medications and also hardened waste-matter imprisoned in the body. All this had complicated his condition, making recovery difficult.

On day four, the NG tube was still slowly removing the toxic matter clogged in his system. When the tube was finally removed, Aditya was still tired, weak and experiencing intense pain. The nauseous feeling persisted. Earlier, every six hours he had been on Reglan, an anti-nausea medication, with morphine or Vicodin and some other painkillers. The heavy pain medication was tapered down so that the toxic build-up was gradually controlled.

By night, a tired Aditya, who had been without any food for the past few days, suffered unbearable pain, and the nausea kept him in extreme discomfort. To give him relief and get him to sleep through the night, the nurse gave him Phenergan. This anti-nausea medication was supposed to help him feel better.

Believing that there would be a lull that night, I settled down to sleep. The past few days had been tiring, and my body was crying for a good rest.

It was close to midnight when I was woken up by noises. Aditya was sitting and commanding his friends, calling out the names of those who had visited him earlier in the evening. It was scary, since he was alone, but his eyes were wide open, with a glint that suggested he could be suffering psychological disorders or showing signs of paranormal phenomena.

Shocked at the vision before me, I asked him in a harsh voice to wake him from his stupor, 'Aditya, what's happened? Who are you talking to?'

As if to confirm to myself, I said softly, 'There's no one here.'

He continued to keep up his line of questioning, the shadows from his bed-light adding mystery to the setting. I stood up, frozen with shock by this sudden change in Aditya. I was stupefied and did not know what to do. Time came to a standstill as my eyes continued to gather the scene before me, and my mind captured its nuances.

Panic-stricken, with my reflexes held back by this shocking sight, I walked out of the room soundlessly but with quick strides, wanting to get help. I was aware of the hollowness inside my stomach, and the strange glint in Aditya's eyes.

At the nurses' station I spoke in a complete daze to the first nurse in sight. Incoherently, I told her that Aditya was probably hallucinating. A nurse rushed in, followed by the designated room nurse. After checking him completely, shining a flashlight in his eyes, and getting him to respond to light as it moved in different directions, I was told that his condition was a result of the side effects of the drug and that it would wear off soon.

After the nurses left, the sudden silence left me with strange broodings. There was a deep fear of being caught in another world, return from which would be another battle. Inside me I could feel the tremor building, and, under the influence of such disturbing thoughts, I made a call at an unearthly hour, nearing two o'clock at night, to Dhananjay. I needed to communicate with someone.

With controlled emotions, which the voice barely disguised, I spoke, 'Dhana, I feel as if I am losing Aditya. Two days back it was the excessive vomiting. Now, half an hour back, he started muttering nonsensical things.'

Dhananjay was awakened from deep sleep. He reacted slowly, after pausing for a few minutes, saying, 'Amma, what happened?'

'It's a medication to relieve pain and control nausea . . . but Aditya reacted . . . it was so bad.'

With the information sinking in, he said, 'Amma . . . shall I fly down tomorrow?'

I told him, with whatever courage I could muster, 'They think the effects will wear off soon. But I just wanted to let you know . . . I am feeling so bad.'

Gathering my wits, I added, 'It's okay . . . no need to come in a hurry.' I realised the folly of undertaking any trip to Los Angeles at that point. It would mean leave from work, which he could use effectively when it was needed.

'Let's wait and see. I think it may be all right by morning.

Try and get some sleep. Will call you later . . .'

I called Srini in Dubai and disturbed his peace at work. He spoke with a calmness that I knew was a façade that he wore while I was nursing our son. Srini was sorely hurt. His kid son going from one health problem to another, with never a peaceful moment, shook him. But all of us had learned to stay strong.

Next morning, a young intern came to us with some research she had done. She said, 'We checked for the bacteria that brought about the infection. It has been identified as a gram-negative bacilli, which is technically known as pasteurella.'

After a few minutes, she asked Aditya, 'Are you in contact with any animals? Did you do something like go to the zoo? I can't understand how else you would have contracted this bacterium.'

It dawned on Aditya what had given him this serious infection. Sheepishly, but without regret, he talked of Gamow and said he had felt her tug at the catheter the previous night. Thereafter he had locked her in the closet. The problem identified, treatment for pasteurella began.

In a few days, Aditya was better and was discharged from the hospital.

He recovered, took a strong hold of his health, organised his diet, and became more careful in setting up the dialysis. This did not stop him from engaging himself with weekend trips and camps with his complete entourage—dialysis machine, a dolly with supplies, and the paraphernalia of clamps, disconnect caps, mask, medication hand wash, and his bag of medications.

At other times he faced problems of mechanical failures when the cycler machine stubbornly refused to start or gave way in the middle of a session. The twenty-four-hour technical support was helpful at most times.

There were many times when the cycler machine did not budge, and we had to resort to using the microwave to warm the manual dialsate supplies to do manual exchanges. The fear of being stranded without getting dialysed is something that is unimaginable.

Reflections
Peritonitis is known to be very painful. But with pasteurella infecting the peritoneum cavity, Aditya had experienced a far more dangerous type of infection caused by contact with animal saliva. Curing the infection took every talent under a doctor's cap and Aditya's own determination.

The nightmare over, we were able to look at options for long-term solutions.

Time for a Decision

Aditya's episode with peritonitis made us sit up.

The various hospitalisations left a dent in our confidence, shattered our peace, and took a huge toll on our energies. At constant guard since Aditya was fifteen, I had no place to bury my head when my own heart grew heavy. The worst was the pasteurella, which was avoidable but happened as part of the life we had chosen, while the others were incidents that happened at every turn during our passage through kidney failure. Very early, fear had set in, making us guarded, and we picked up cues quickly to take action. That was fortunate.

The emergency admissions, the repeated surgeries, the machine failures, are all expected events in every kidney patient's life, some experienced more intensely, others less. What one cannot anticipate is when exactly things will go wrong.

If the dialysis is insufficient because of machine failures or excess fluid load, the discomfort is unimaginable. These experiences remain with the patient and cannot find expression.

But this incident gave us an opportunity to review the status of Aditya's health and find other means for his survival. Persistent health problems kept us worried. Strong medicines like morphine and anti-nausea medications, with their side effects, affected his health in many ways. I had watched him approach end-of-life situations so many times that it became necessary to get Aditya ready for a transplant. His refusal to look in that direction was something that I needed to work on.

Srini had earlier expressed his desire to donate a kidney. His blood tests had revealed that his albumin was well within normal limits, which had surprised Dr Gandhi. Further tests were needed to be sure that donating a kidney would not be detrimental to Srini's health. He had to do the twenty-four-hour urine test for protein levels and have the fundus of his eye checked for any indications of retinopathy. While we were having discussions to move Srini's evaluation forward, Dhananjay vetoed it and renewed his offer of over-a-decade-ago. As the elder of the two brothers, who was involved in every problem that surfaced with

Aditya, it was the most natural step.

Reflections

Dhananjay made the decision to donate his kidney. As usual, my reaction was slow and late. I was confused. I was torn between feeling happy for one son, while I felt a little guilty over my lack of emotion in allowing Dhananjay to part with his kidney.

A mother can never show partiality, and here I was being put to the test. Dhananjay took it in his stride. There was no time for tears. I knew I had no reason to worry, as a person can live a long life with a single kidney . . . how often had I said it before? Yet there was some restlessness; somewhere below, in my female heart, there was a tug. After all, it was my son . . . Dhananjay . . . my first treasure. Was I doing the right thing?

I also knew we had no other option. Srini was nearing sixty, and the combination of age and diabetes was certainly on the wrong side for a transplant. Aditya was not willing to let his father go through this.

So, amidst differing viewpoints played out by my overactive brain, I selfishly pursued the option that presented itself . . . now with the faith that God would lead us to the end of our tribulations.

In his own proactive manner, Aditya had a few years earlier approached hospitals such as USC Medical Center and Beverly Hills' Cedars Sinai Medical Center to get on the transplant list with the official organ transplant body, United Network for Organ Sharing.

Conversations with a social worker at Cedars Sinai Medical Center gave us hope. It began with an evaluation of Aditya's health. He was listed on the National Transplant List in December 2008 after the process was completed.

Our first real progress was in February 2009 when Dhananjay was called in for his evaluation. It began with blood tests to check HLA, apart from the renal profile.

Aditya was highly sensitised from his earlier transplant. The antibodies from my body cells, as well as his, would not withstand the trials of a fresh transplant. Till 2004, patients who were highly sensitised could not undergo a transplant for fear of rejection of the transplanted organ.

All the experimentation and testing at Cedars Sinai led to the FDA finally approving the IVIG (Intravenous Immunoglobulin) protocol that was developed under the leadership of Dr Stanley Jordan, director of the Division of Nephrology at Cedars Sinai. For the first time, with the IVIG desensitisation protocol, a patient who was highly sensitised due to pregnancy, blood transfusion, a previous transplant or any other reason could be made eligible for a transplant.

Aditya was recommended for IVIG infusion with dialysis, followed by Rituxan therapy, a second IVIG infusion with dialysis, and a last IVIG infusion post transplant. This aimed to reduce the antibodies and to secure the kidney from possible rejection.

The treatment would be spread over four weeks, with the first one scheduled on 7 May.

Dhananjay underwent tests too, including EKG, chest X-ray, renal sonography, and angiography. The left kidney was approved for the transplant. But the meetings with the hospital's donor team proved to be strenuous. He had to satisfy them of his genuine desire to donate the kidney. This was part of the prerequisite for getting approved as a live-donor transplant. His medical reports, too, were reviewed in great detail to protect his health as a donor and to safeguard his future.

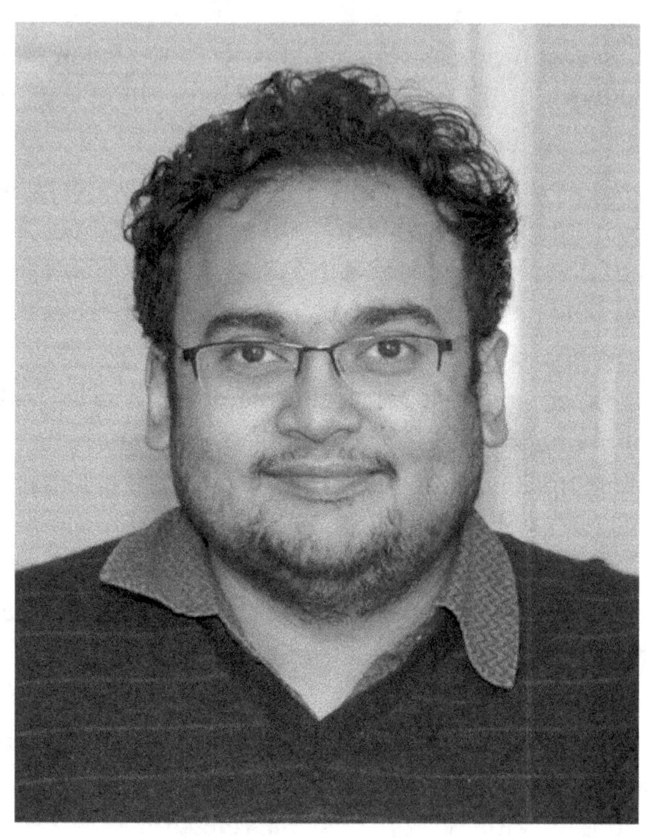

A relaxed Dhananjay after clearing medical tests

The Sunrise on Our Horizon

June 2009

The transplant was scheduled for 9 June 2009.

It was ten years and two months after the first transplant. Our world suddenly seemed to be blessed. The sun rose from the east, as on any other day, but it shone brighter to light our path to life beyond.

The surgery was at Cedars Sinai, Beverly Hills. We arrived at the hospital at five o'clock in the morning. The registration had been done during our last visit when Aditya had his second IVIG infusion. So we had to report to Admissions, from where we were guided to the sixth floor for the surgery.

Dhananjay was taken in first, at seven o'clock.

Reflections

Srini and I were full of worry. We said silent prayers for our brave son who had suddenly wiped the lines of worry from our foreheads by offering his kidney. Concern for him and his future played in our minds. After all, we are parents, and in spite of all that science tells us, our hearts will always give us a different signal.

For parents, every child holds our attention in a unique way. It appears that our heart has flexible compartments for each offspring, to hold deposits of love, prayers for success, space for pride, and anything that brings them happiness. Above all, we have a huge capacity to bear their pain, in a measure that cannot be interpreted in terms of volume. The size of each slot gets expanded on the basis of need. There is no way that one can explain logically why parents feel differently at different times.

Dhananjay showed us his commitment and played the role of the older brother with great composure. This was his first hospitalisation ... why was I not running around and fussing?

I watched the whole replay of the transplant like a spectator. My only thought was ... what next? Or, this should be done ... a very objective view for an otherwise emotional mother! That was the change that had happened to me silently through the phase of Aditya's hospitalisations. My sisters applauded Dhananjay's act as one not many a sibling would do. I heard their feelings with quiet acceptance, without exhibiting pride. Such pride would lower the relevance of Dhananjay's generosity.

I knew Dhananjay wanted me to simply love him for this act. I did just that. Within me I could feel that the compartments for love and pride for him had grown in size.

The surgeon met us after an hour to give us the status on the surgery. The kidney had been removed, and Dhananjay was in stable condition. Aditya was taken in nearly an hour after Dhananjay's surgery.

Srini, Dhananjay's friend Anshul, and I waited anxiously. Between coffee breaks we received information on Aditya's progress in surgery. Finally the surgeon came out of the operating room to inform us that Dhananjay's kidney had started producing urine in Aditya's body while still on the operation table.

That was pure music to our ears.

Getting the surgery done at Cedars Sinai was a great experience. The whole process was well planned and well coordinated, thanks to years of experience doing kidney transplants, most of them successful. The staff and doctors were systematic and professional, and that was how they managed to stay on top of the charts for organ transplants. At each stage we were involved with information pouring out of the operating room. We were made part of the process. They showed an understanding of how we were vulnerable and how every bit of information made it better for us.

We visited each of our sons while in the recovery room. Dhananjay was out earlier, so we visited him several times. He was under the effects of anaesthesia, and gradually when he showed signs of recovery, he was in intense pain. In the recovery room his vital signs were monitored and he was watched for any complication in the post-surgery stage. Recovery rooms are equipped with oxygen masks and any issues with breathing or circulation can be treated at the early recovery stage, thereby avoiding major complications. Staff is available to oversee the patients while in recovery and they keep the patient comfortable.

By early evening Dhananjay and Aditya were allotted rooms. The rooms were on different floors and across the landing from each other.

Dhananjay was advised to walk around on day one itself, so he was up and about, walking down the passage to Aditya's room. Walking soon after surgery would improve the recovery process. It would help in reducing the effects of the anaesthesia and increase energy levels.

Aditya's life changed with his starting immunosuppressant drugs and a battery of medications, including steroids.

Dhananjay faced acute pain but managed it well with medications like Vicodin that gave him relief for a few hours. Srini and I kept running between the rooms trying to help in the best way possible. Anshul was very helpful in keeping Dhananjay company when we were busy.

Dhananjay was discharged in three days. I got great help from my niece Urmil who came from Houston to engage the two recovering patients with conversation and divert attention from their aches and pains. With her assistance, we managed fresh, nutritious food and basic home-nursing care to bring them back to their feet.

Aditya came home five days after surgery. The nursing staff conducted a workshop on management of medications. A seven-day organiser was advised for filling medicines and an alert call so that medicines were taken at an appointed time.

Charts had to be maintained for blood pressure, and the dosage of medications would be tapered down as Aditya's condition improved over the next few weeks.

Standard reporting formats were handed over.

The immunosuppressant that was prescribed was Prograf, along with the steroid prednisolone. These drugs were known to have side effects, of which the most immediate for concern were sugar levels in blood and cholesterol levels. This could be managed through diet, and if that was not possible, medications would be advised.

Our first task was to provide a nutritious, high-protein, low-carbohydrate, low-fat diet.

So we worked on meals, bringing in low-fat cream cheese, adding berries for dessert, and relying heavily on tofu and soy beans in the main course and snacks with edamame and plenty of vegetables and salads. Bread was now mainly wholewheat, as against white bread while on dialysis.

Life changed again. Now new medications and new management of health and diet engaged our attention. Though it was a path taken before, the to and fro on diet, medications and water consumption (limited during dialysis and not less than three litres in post-transplant condition) meant we thought of it as 'new' so that we could learn it anew.

The weekly laboratory work, follow-up with the doctors, the last IVIG infusion and medication planning took a major part of our time during the weeks that followed. Aditya showed good progress, and the doctors were happy. Dhananjay resumed work a fortnight after the surgery.

At the end of July, when I visited him in California's South Bay, he was neck-deep in a major project. Still weak after the surgery, a certain happiness illuminated his face whenever he heard that his younger brother was doing well.

That is the prize of giving, be it a part of your body or a part of your wealth. Happiness comes with the act of giving, the act of knowing that you have changed someone's life for the better; happiness is the act of loving life and living.

Aditya's Professional Life

On 14 May, Aditya defended his research in front of a team of experts including his advisor, Dr Stephan Haas. The defense was accepted, and he became Dr Aditya Raghavan. The graduation ceremony was on 5 June 2009, four days before his second transplant.

Two months later we drove across the country northward, through Las Vegas, Yellowstone National Park, the Grand Canyon, and through Banff and Jasper National Parks to Edmonton, Canada. Aditya had accepted a post-doctorate fellowship at Alberta University. Since his graduation he was full of plans on how he would enjoy life in Alberta; how this post-doctorate under Dr Kevin Beach was an excellent break. Dr Stephan Haas had introduced him to Beach.

It was in Aditya's nature to accept everything wholeheartedly. So also it was with the move to Edmonton. He talked about the country, the parks and natural life. Everything in life looked interesting now, with a new kidney to help him along.

He registered himself at the university's hospital and is now under the excellent care of Dr Murray.

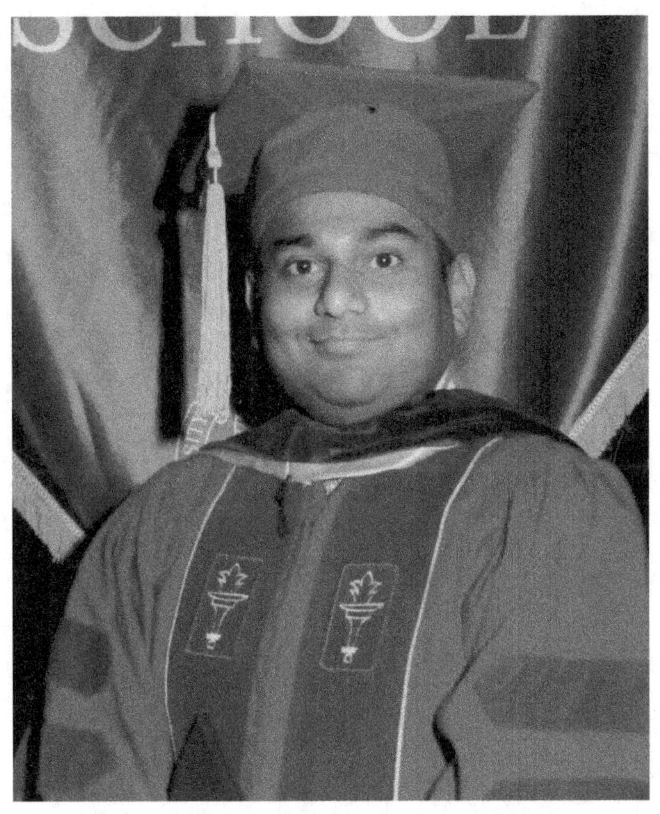

Graduating with a doctorate in physics

Some weekends, one can see Aditya's car taking a turn on Saskatchewan Drive, heading toward the famed Jasper National Park, Canada's largest national park. The trips generally are inspired by his passion for nature, wildlife and photography.

The excitement in life continues. It is new friends now, a new life and new ways to find joy! Trips to the United States to meet family and friends, seminars and conferences, learning to speak French, music on the guitar and keyboard, and photography are keeping life exciting. Cooking has reached another level, as it involves more grilling and baking.

Aditya takes full advantage of this phase in life. His mind is never idle, as every day he has new ideas and plans for his life ahead, both personal and professional. Notwithstanding it all, he has come to live life for the moment. No whisper of any dark days in the past, but walking into a future fuelled by aspirations.

Addendum

Aditya Raghavan was on a post doctoral fellowship with University of Alberta, Canada when he set out to the prairies to discover a whole new world beyond physics. Big Addie (as he's now known in his friend circles) is now an artisan cheese maker, forager and is cofounder of "Danda Food Project" which does curative dining and does interesting pop up dinners in Bandra, Mumbai. He has travelled far away from academics.

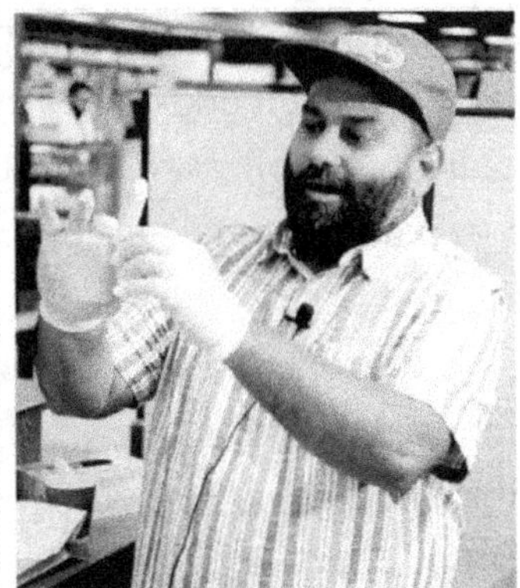

Recently he was awarded by ASASA for Culinary Arts for bringing regional farm cheeses into forefront, in India and overseas.

Afterword

There is so much happiness when a doctor/nurse proves himself/herself and brings us relief from our illness; there is, equally, insurmountable sorrow when their action or inaction causes damage to or leads to the death of a patient. The doctor, then, becomes the target of our deep hatred.

Everyone's experiences with medical treatment and doctors are not the same. It is just as it is in life: some people seem to have all the luck, and some do not meet with so much good fortune. It is also the same with the services we receive. When we get a raw deal, it is natural for us to express our feelings and react with anger. And when it involves the life of a human being, it crosses the threshold level and the anger is justified.

On retrospect, it is for each of us to determine what went wrong.

Doctors are remarkable people, dedicating their lives to the service of humankind. Their education and training have made them experts. But we should remember that although they have great expertise, having earlier handled many challenging medical cases, they may be unsuccessful in treating some patients.

Doctors are just as human as we are. So we must begin with that real statement.

Then break down cases of failure.

Was the doctor not qualified? What was his or her previous record in the cases he or she had handled? Did you check on that? Did you have the option to change the doctor? Did you put complete faith in the doctor? Did you follow all the instructions on dos and don'ts? Did the doctor do all that was possible or was he or she negligent?

If you have done your homework and selected your doctor, is he or she still to blame?

If the answer is yes . . . consider this.

How often have we broken a precious glass? Can we remember how often we had burnt food, spoilt a dress, lost an important document, banged a car while in reverse gear, or accidentally closed the door on a child's hand? All these accidents happen in spite of exercising utmost care. If we make an excuse that we made a mistake and that we were careful, but somehow things did not happen as desired . . . can we consider that the doctor also made a mistake? After all, his or her job also involves mundane day-to-day tasks of scrubbing, making a cut for a surgery, closing the opening with surgical sutures . . . sometimes he or she can make a mistake. So can he or she say, 'sorry' and get away with it? Can we forgive? He or she made a mistake that was unintentional. It is only when the doctor is consistently negligent that harsh steps need to be taken.

In cases of patients with life-threatening diseases, it is particularly true that it is a matter of understanding that the chance for survival is not totally in the hands of the doctor.

Our experiences during the incidents when Aditya faced peritonitis told us clearly that there is much more than meets the eye.

It is God's will that things happen how they do. After all, doctors are far less capable than God.

There is so much pressure on doctors to perform and cure every patient, see that every surgery is successful and to be patient and kind with their patients. They must be God's priciest creations—unique, infallible, and almost as perfect as a computer.

Unfortunately accidents happen even with doctors. With every disease, from kidney failure to cancer to HIV, one point needs acceptance: not all patients are the same.

Each patient needs special treatment, as his or her medical condition is different. The dosage for chemotherapy is different for different kinds of cancer. For ovarian cancer it could be twenty-four hours or more of chemotherapy treatment, while for breast cancer it may be a few hours. Nothing is standardised. It depends also on the stage of the cancer. For kidney patients, everything depends heavily on lab work, diet, and medications, with all their side effects.

These illnesses are a part of us due to the combined effects of our luck, the quality of life, the treatments we take, among several other factors.. If we can accept this, our doctors can work with our full confidence bestowed on them.

Remember, doctors are ordinary human beings. Let us leave them that way.

After all, success and failure are the outcome of the factor that one calls 'luck'. But it is fate that seals it all.

People say that treatment should be timely. In my opinion we should learn to rise to the occasion. In both Vasundhara's medical history and Aditya's, we decided to act without losing time procrastinating.

When it was decided that Vasundhara would donate her kidney, she was detected with breast cancer. No time was lost in curing her of breast cancer and making the kidney available for transplant.

In 2006, when the kidney failed a second time, the situation was tackled by starting haemodialysis and later peritoneal dialysis. All this was advised by the attending doctors. We took time to decide on a second transplant; when Dhananjay offered to donate his kidney, and the tests showed there was a match, we could proceed.

It is important that the family works in sync and understands the need to take treatments without delay.

From Aditya's medical history, it became evident that for end-stage kidney failures, kidney transplant was possibly the best solution.

However, there are challenges in getting a willing donor with a matching kidney, proper hospitals that can successfully do the transplant with good post-transplant care, and the patient taking enough precautions to save the transplanted kidney. Most important, availability of money or insurance to meet expenses related to medicines and any treatment required post transplant is necessary.

This calls for a proper health-care policy by governments, including having world-class hospitals and subsidised/free medical facilities.

SRINIVAS RAGHAVAN

Acknowledgements

To our most valued supporters—doctors and medical professionals.

Dr Bhupendra V. Gandhi

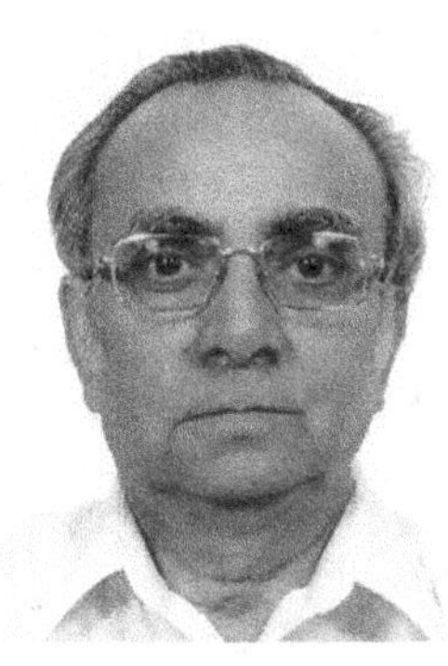

Aditya's early understanding of the medical aspects of his health came through close interactions with Dr Bhupendra V. Gandhi. Mumbai's leading nephrologist, widely recognised in India for his extensive knowledge and expertise, showed Aditya how to be completely in charge of his health care.

The doctor's educational background as a fellow in nephrology and his experiences while practising as a consulting nephrologist at Detroit's kidney centre; training at Peter Brent Brigham Hospital (the hospital that was responsible for the first successful human-to-human kidney transplant, in 1954); and thereafter, setting up departments of nephrology (handling dialysis and renal transplants) at Mumbai's three major institutions—Breach Candy Hospital,

D. Balabhai Nanavati Hospital and Bhatia Hospital—created in us a trust and confidence in his capabilities. Appreciating his work, we hold him in the highest esteem.

His deep involvement with patient cases, his intelligence and his excellence in handling patient-doctor relationship need special mention. We know that patients across the world rely on his knowledgeable medical advice and get treated.

The National Kidney Foundation India, the Indian Society of Nephrology and the Bombay Nephrology Group benefit from his active involvement. Recently, he was bestowed with a Lifetime Achievement Award for his contributions in the field of nephrology, by the Madras

Kidney Trust and Hypertension Foundation. We are proud of his achievements and contributions in creating programmes for awareness of renal disease and his recognition both on his home turf and overseas for his numerous publications.

Late Dr Arun Kurkure

Aditya's first transplant became a reality after Dr Arun Kurkure gave me the most appropriate treatment to cure me of cancer. Our appreciation for his efforts is overwhelming.

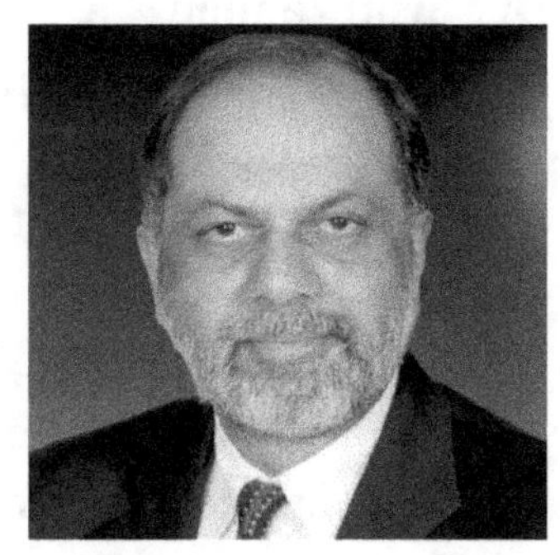

With a degree in surgery- oncology and a certificate course in hospital management, Dr Kurkure started services for bringing relief to cancer patients. His education, excellent work skills and humane approach to patients and their families bought him repute as he worked his way up at the prestigious Breach Candy Hospital and Medical Centre as a breast cancer surgeon and gynaecological oncologist.

He grew professionally by introducing the hub-and-spoke model ('Think globally and act locally') to the future activities of the UICC (the International Union of Cancer). He had a significant impact on cancer control in India and throughout the world. He has contributed greatly to the mission of the UICC as an executive committee member and through his involvement with the 2006 UICC World Cancer Congress Programme Executive Committee.

His association, in a managerial capacity, with top national and international NGOs for cancer prevention has given him the chance to grow and widen the scope of his service to reach the most distant parts of the world. He is leading several projects related to his field, on patient rehabilitation and support systems for patients, and his deep involvement in activities related to cancer-control strategies set him apart as a man of great purpose.

Dr Shruti Tandan

Shruti was a friend, philosopher and guide to Aditya. When his life changed dramatically, her constant support kept him centred. She entered the famed KEM Hospital and SGS Medical College for her degree in medicine. She was a multi- talented teenager, possessing the unique quality of managing all her talents, 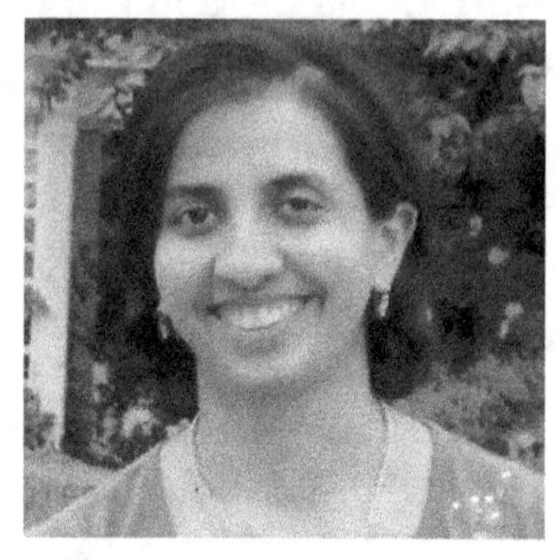 nurturing them and giving them an outlet now and then. Her intelligence, creative thinking, liveliness, leadership qualities, and, above all, the spirit to conquer, set her apart.

Her decision to bring her humanness to the forefront by pursuing a career in medicine made us proud. She has made service to humanity her mission, keeping under wraps her other exceptional talents.

After a postgraduation degree in internal medicine at AIIMS, New Delhi, and a short stint at Lilavati Hospital, she was chosen to further her career and was awarded a fellowship by the National Board in Critical Care Medicine. She moved towards doing some cherished work at Mumbai's Jaslok Hospital as a full-time intensivist.

Our memories of her early medical consultancy, whenAditya was detected with kidney failure, will remain fresh for all times to come.

Dr Mohammad Akmal

One of USC's reputed and experienced nephrologists, Dr Mohammad Akmal influenced Aditya positively while he pursued his post-doctorate programme in the United States. The doctor's unique approach to treatments and sharing medical information benefited Aditya in managing his health better. Akmal's greatest attribute 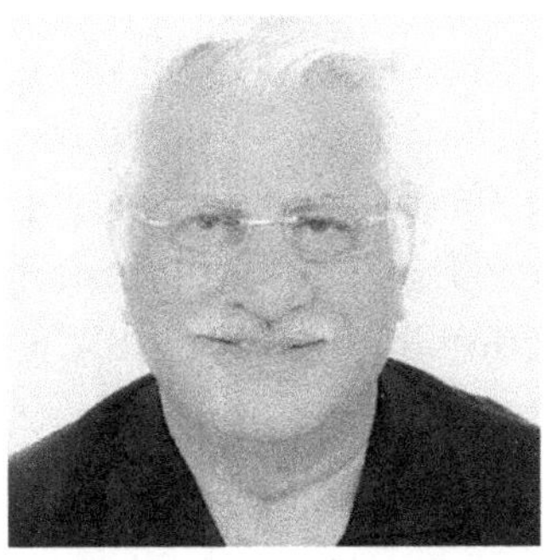 is his humaneness. His kindness and warm-heartedness endears him to his patients and associates. He has an extraordinary capability of adopting well-considered treatment measures in resolving issues. We have respect for and implicit trust in him.

A fellow in nephrology from Ohio's Christ Hospital, Cincinnati and Los Angeles County Medical Center in California, he was appointed as a professor of medicine at the USC Keck School of Medicine, medical director of the dialysis programme, and a director of the USC/DaVita Kidney Center. Professionally he excels in service of his patients, and demonstrates great sensitivity in treating with appropriate attention people with differing levels of seriousness of the disease.

His service to several renal communities in leadership capacities such as President of the Medical Advisory Board and Chairman of the Board of Directors, Southern California National Kidney Foundation, and Chairman of the Board of Directors, Southern California Renal Disease Council, Inc. Network 18, confirms his commitment to help a larger section of humankind. We take great pride in his accomplishments, and our appreciation for him is immeasurable.

He is the author of over sixty-five scientific publications and chapters, and several meritorious awards have come his way. He has received the Spirit of Nephrology Award from the Southern California National Kidney Foundation and the 'Dr Pepper Award' from DaVita Inc. (Wild West Division).

Other major recognitions Dr Akmal has received include 'Man of The Year in Medicine and Healthcare, 2008' (American Biographical Institute), 'America's Top Physicians, 2008' (Consumer Research Council of America), 'Super Doctor, Southern California 2008' (Key Professional Media, Inc.), and 'Professional of the Year, 2007' (the Global Directory of Who's Who).

Dr Mustafa Ahmed

My association with Dr Mustafa Ahmed, at Dubai's Welcare Hospital, began in November 1996, while I was trying to arrange the Christmas vacation dialysis for Aditya. At that time I learned that, while dialysis was being offered to patients, there was no transplant programme in the UAE.

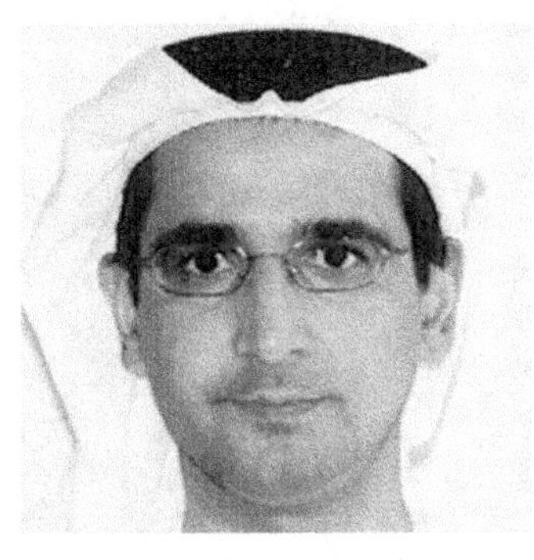

Exactly two years later, I was unprepared to hear Dr Ahmed speak with suppressed excitement on a subject close to his heart—the ten transplants conducted in the country. It was music to my ears. I was able to interview a few of his UAE patients, whose cases will be available to you in our next publication.

Dr Mustafa Ahmed, a UAE national, graduated from London's King's College and was drawn into nephrology. His interest in the field grew while investigating abnormal cellular transport systems in uraemia in Oxford and Santiago. He has working experience from the Middlesex Institute of Nephro-Urology, the renal unit attached to the King's College Hospital and the Guy's and St Thomas' Hospital, one of the largest transplant centres in the UK.

His doctorate on nocturnal polyuria won him a national award from the UK Renal Association. He has conducted major studies on live related/unrelated transplantation, transplantation across blood-group barriers, and SPK (simultaneous kidney pancreas transplantation) and was involved with London's largest study on 'transplant tourism'. He is now serving leading hospitals in the UAE, with its diverse population and different health-care needs. As an avid campaigner for transplantation within the boundaries of good ethical practice, he had formed a team that carried out the first successful living related liver and renal transplants in Zayed Military Hospital.

My association with the reputed doctor helped in my appreciation

of how work in the area of kidney transplants has grown in the UAE
in such a short time.

Mr K. Raghuram

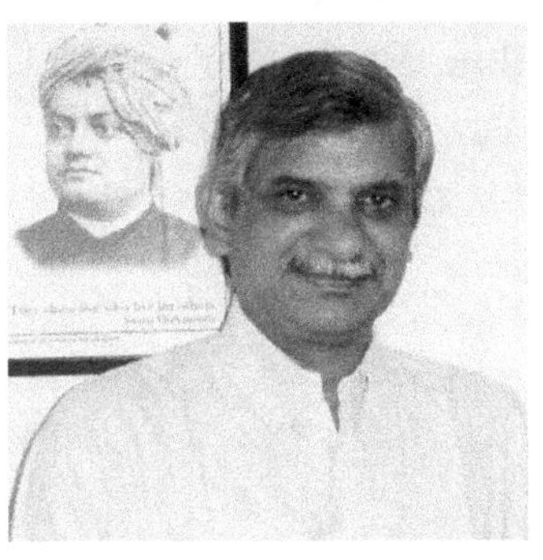

In 2006, when Aditya's kidney was rejected, I came into contact with Mr Raghuram, who was serving MOHAN (the Multi Organ Harvesting Aid Network), representing the Hyderabad office. He shared with me how cadaver transplants were made possible through his organisation and his personal efforts. Their work interested me and our association grew strong with mutual respect for each other. Coincidently, after both Raghuram and his wife Lalitha became part of MOHAN, destiny placed them in a situation when the decision to donate their son's organs became immediate. Their nineteen-year-old-son met with a fatal car accident and was declared brain dead. They decided to donate his eyes and other organs.

As have other organ-donation agencies, MOHAN faces multiple challenges. Corneal transplants were huge in numbers, but obtaining permission for the retrieval of other organs posed problems. Understanding how Western countries have achieved significant success in this area was critical, and soon they started seeing more opportunities for transplants.

MOHAN's teams have consistently worked towards creating awareness through workshops, campaigns and signature drives to make organ donation part of an application for a driving license and/or to create permanent account numbers for income taxes, known popularly as a PAN card, and by enlisting brand ambassadors for promoting organ donations. These are a few of the organisation's initiatives.

MOHAN has been instrumental in spearheading changes in legislation through dialogues with the Government of India. These changes mean that more people will have the opportunity to donate organs posthumously.

For an emerging country, organising organ transplant ethically is its biggest challenge in an environment where organ trade had flourished before.

Glossary of Technical Terms

Access: Access is created for entering the bloodstream so that dialysis can be done. In the case of haemodialysis, a fistula acts as the access.

Anaemia: If a person feels weak, breathless and less energetic, it may be indicative of being anaemic. When the blood has a shortage of red cells, anaemia occurs. For improvement, iron and erythropoietin will be needed.

Artery: Artery is the blood vessel that carries blood from the heart to the rest of the body.

Bladder: From the kidney, the urine goes into the organ known as the bladder, before being released from the body.

Blood cells: The blood is made up of microscopic cells that are known as blood cells. Blood cells consist of red and white cells and platelets.

Blood group: Our blood can be classified into four main groups: A, B, AB, and O. The classification system is based on hereditary conditions dictating the availability of certain antigens in the cells. Generally blood and organ donations are based on the match of the blood group between the donor and recipient.

Blood pressure: When the blood passes through the arteries, it exerts a certain level of pressure against their walls. This pressure is measured as blood pressure. Blood pressure is an important determinant for many surgeries and indicates the health condition of a person.

- Normal blood pressure: is 120/80 millimeters of mercury (mm Hg) or less
- Prehypertension: between 120/80mm Hg and 139/89 mm Hg
High: more than 140/90 mm Hg
- If your age is over sixty-five, blood pressure up to 150/90 mm Hg can be considered normal

Bone marrow: In some bones, such as hip and thigh bones, there is a soft tissue in the hollow, interior portion, which is known as bone marrow. New blood cells get created here.

Cadaveric transplant: This is a transplant surgery done with a kidney or other organ removed from a person who is brain dead or has died in an accident.

Calcium: This is a mineral salt that strengthens the bones.

Catheter: A catheter is a flexible plastic tube that is inserted when access to the body's interior is needed.

Cholesterol: This is a measure of the level of fat in the bloodstream. There is a risk of having heart diseases or strokes if the blood shows a high cholesterol value. Though high cholesterol is dangerous, the levels can be reduced with diet and drugs.

Creatinine: When muscles are used, a waste substance known as creatinine is produced. A blood test is used to measure creatinine, and it indicates whether or not the kidney is functioning normally.

The normal values for creatinine are: 0.6-1.2 milligrams per deciliter (mg/dL).

Crossmatch: The crossmatch is different from tissue-type or blood-group match. Crossmatch is a blood test to check for the existence of any antibodies. Antibodies normally help the body fight infection and would react with the donor kidney. High levels of antibodies may lead to rejection, even if it is a good tissue-type match.

Crossmatch: is done by mixing a sample of the recipient's blood with cells from the donor. If the recipient's blood starts attacking the donor cells, there is the likelihood that the kidney will be rejected.

Dehydration: The body is dehydrated when there is insufficient water in the body for its proper functioning.

Diabetes: When high levels of glucose are found in the blood and urine, a condition popularly known as diabetes is said to be the problem. This happens because of poor functioning of the pancreas. The world over, people with diabetes are at high risk for kidney failure.

Dialyser: A dialysis machine has a filtering unit known as a dialyser, which removes waste products and excess water from the blood.

Dialysis: The process of removing the waste products and excess water from the blood when the kidneys cease to perform this function properly is known as dialysis.

Diuretic drugs: Medicines administered to increase urine outputs are called diuretics.

Donor: A person who donates an organ, blood, or tissue to another person is known as a donor.

Dry weight: The body weight after dialysis is called a dry weight. The weight is without excess fluid in the lungs or in the tissues.

Erythropoietin (EPO): When the kidney functions properly, this is a hormone that it produces, along with several others. This hormone stimulates the bone marrow to produce red blood cells. But when the kidney fails, the person may become anaemic if lower levels of red blood cells get produced. In such a situation, EPO injections may be given to perform the hormone's function.

Fistula: In order to provide access to the bloodstream for haemodialysis, a vein may be enlarged surgically. This access is called a fistula.

Fluid overload: This is excess water in the body caused by excess consumption of water, or not being able to pass enough urine.

Glomerular Filtration Rate (GFR): The GFR shows exactly how much kidney function is left. Though measuring the level of creatinine in the blood helps in estimating the kidney function, it is not very accurate. If the GFR falls below 30, the person should see a kidney disease specialist—a nephrologist. It is time to learn about treatments for kidney failure like dialysis or kidney transplant. If the GFR falls below 15, the person needs to start treatment immediately.

Haemodialysis (HD): A more popular form of dialysis for blood purification. The blood is cleaned outside the body by a dialysis machine, which takes between three and four hours to finish the process.

Haemoglobin: The red blood cells have haemoglobin, which carries oxygen to all parts of the body.

Hormone: This is a substance that acts as a chemical messenger in the body, controlling various bodily functions.

Ideal body weight: An ideal body weight is determined based on the age, sex and height of the person. This is the expected range for people falling within that group.

Immune system: Everybody has an immune system that protects the body from infections and foreign bodies. In the case of a person who has had a transplant, the system is suppressed by medication so that it does not reject the foreign organ. The immune system therefore works less effectively.

Immunosuppressant drugs: These are drugs prescribed to transplant patients to make the immune system less effective so that it does not fight the foreign body, which is the transplanted kidney or other organ. Immunosuppressant drugs are required to protect the kidney from being rejected.

Malnutrition: This condition occurs because of weight loss, due to lower consumption of food providing protein and energy.

Nasogastric tube: This is normally called the NG tube. It is made of a flexible material of rubber or plastic. The tube, used to put substances, including nutrients, into the stomach, is inserted through the nose and then through the oesophagus into the stomach when a patient is unable to eat or drink by mouth.

Sometimes the tube is used to remove contents from the stomach, including air, small solid objects, fluid and other toxic substances that cannot be removed normally through the stool.

Nephritis: This is an inflammation of the kidneys.

Nephron: The kidney is made up of many small units called nephrons, which do the filtering and balance fluid in the body.

Oedema: This is an abnormal accumulation of water in the body. If the water is accumulated in the lungs, it is called pulmonary oedema.

Omentum: The omentum hangs like a curtain from the bottom of the stomach, right in front of the intestines. It is like a sheet of fatty tissue that stores body fat, and it grows as more fat is accumulated. It contains germ-fighting cells that can migrate to the abdomen and helps to seal it off. The omentum therefore protects the abdomen from infections. For the surgeon the omentum acts as a handy tool—something like a biological duct tape. Portions of the omentum may be used as a graft in cut areas to heal them. The omentum can be also a source of problems. When its blood supply is interrupted, there are symptoms of severe pain and tenderness that can wrongly be diagnosed as appendicitis. Another aspect is that when it is enlarged due to high-fat storage, it results in a protruding belly, and the person does not look very pleasing.

Peritoneal dialysis (PD): This form of dialysis uses the peritoneum as a filter. The blood is cleaned inside the person's body, not externally, as in haemodialysis. PD is a home- dialysis programme.

Peritoneum: This is a natural membrane lining the walls of the abdomen.

Peritoneal Cavity: This is the area in the abdomen where the stomach, liver, and bowels are found.

Phosphate: An important substance involved with calcium that accumulates when the kidneys fail.

Phosphate binders: In order to avoid the build-up of phosphate in the blood, phosphate binders are prescribed. They absorb excess phosphorus from the blood.

Platelets: These are a type of blood cell that helps in clotting blood.

Polycystic kidney disease: This kidney disease is hereditary and results because of a problem in kidney development. The kidneys get enlarged and are full of sacs filled with fluid, which are known as cysts. This disease sometimes leads to kidney failure.

Potassium: This mineral is normally present in the blood but has to be maintained at a particular level. Higher or lower levels may cause heart problems.

Protein: This is essential for muscle formation, and the breakdown products are filtered by the kidney. Meat, fish, dairy products and nuts are rich in protein.

Pulmonary oedema: When the lungs get filled with fluid, the resulting condition is known as pulmonary oedema. It results in breathlessness, especially when lying down flat and exercising.

Pyelonephritis: This is a painless inflammation caused by repeated infections, drugs, or other factors. It occurs in the part of the kidneys that is in between filtering units.

Recipient: A person who receives an organ for transplant from a donor.

Rejection: The immune system fights infection and foreign bodies. In the case of a transplant, the organ transplanted is in fact a foreign body. The immune system may attack the organ, leading to rejection.

Renal: It is the term used for kidneys. A renal failure means a failure of the kidneys.

Satellite haemodialysis unit: A unit that is located away from the main hospital renal unit and provides haemodialysis is known as a satellite unit.

Semi-permeable: A membrane that allows some substances to pass through it is called semi-permeable.

Tenckhoff catheter: In a PD, the catheter that allows access for the dialysis fluid to flow in and out from the peritoneal cavity but is capped off when not in use is known as a Tenckhoff.

Tissue type: A blood test called a tissue-type test is conducted to measure the antigens on the surface of the body and its cells.

Transplant: This surgery is done to plant a new organ, which is donated by someone, into a patient who needs it for survival.

Ultra filtration: This process removes excess water from the blood.

Under dialysis: This happens when dialysis treatment is not sufficient to remove all the water and waste products that are in excess.

Urea: This is one of the main waste products that build up in the blood. In addition to creatinine levels, the levels of urea in the blood are indicative of how the kidneys are functioning.

Ureters: Urine is carried from the kidneys to the bladder through tubes called ureters.

Urethra: The tube that carries urine from the bladder outside the body is called the urethra.

Urine: This is the fluid produced by the kidneys. It is composed of excess water and the toxic waste products that come from food and are not required by the body.

Veins: Blood vessels that carry dark-red-coloured blood are veins. They bring impure blood from different parts of the body to the heart for purification. They have less oxygen and are thinner than arteries.

Use of Information

Over the years, understanding my son's disease at each stage required reading books, different websites and reference material distributed by hospitals, dialysis centres, doctors, social workers and other people involved in this field. With a deep sense of gratitude, I wish to thank the people who enabled our familyto stand up and face the world.

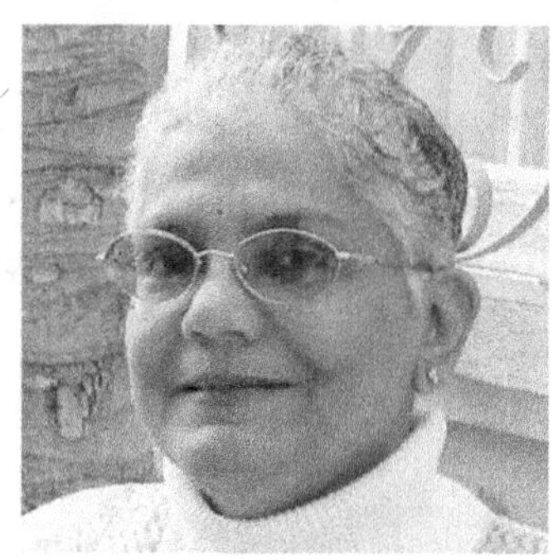

Vasundhara Raghavan

If I have failed to acknowledge any person or organisation, please know that it is purely unintentional. To that organisation or person, I humbly bow and join my hands together in a namaskar, giving full expression of my heartfelt gratitude.

Bibliography

Listed below are some materials I referenced during the process of writing this book. They helped in my understanding and in providing readers information in simple layman's language. I have attempted to write the book with honesty and as simply as possible.

American Heart Association—www.heart.org/HEARTORG

American Kidney Fund—www.kidneyfund.org

American Urology Association—www.auanet.org

Astellas Transplant—www.transplantexperience.com

Cedar-Sinai Medical Center—www.csmc.edu

DaVita—www.davita.com

eMedicineHealth—www.emedicinehealth.com

Healthcommunities.com—www.healthcommunities.com

Kidney School—www.kidneyschool.org

Mayo Clinic—www.mayoclinic.com

MedlinePlus Medical Encyclopedia—www.nlm.nih.gov/
     medlineplus/encyclopedia.html

MedicineNet.com—www.medicinenet.com

National Kidney Foundation, India—www.nkfi.in

National Kidney Foundation, United States—www.kidney.org

National Kidney Foundation,
Southern California— www.kidney.org

National Kidney and Urological Diseases Information
     Clearinghouse—kidney.niddk.nih.gov/kudiseases

Nephrology Channel—www.nephrologychannel.com

Texas Pediatric Surgical Associates—www.pedisurg.com

The Kidney Foundation of Canada—www.kidney.ca

University of Iowa Hospitals and Clinics—www.uihealthcare.com

University of Pennsylvania Health System—www.pennmedicine.org

Acharya, V. N., 'Status of Renal Transplant in India,' *Journal of Postgraduate Medicine* (http://www.jpgmonline.com) 40, no.1 (1994): 158-61.

Stein, Andy, and Wild, Janet, *Kidney Dialysis and Transplants*. London: Class Publishing, 2002.

Garovoy, Marvin R., Guttmann, Ronald D, *Renal Transplantation*. New York: Churchill Livingstone Inc., 1986.

Faris, Michie Hall, *When Your Kidneys Fail*. Southern California: National Kidney Foundation, 1994.

www.ingramcontent.com/pod-product-compliance
Lightning Source LLC
Chambersburg PA
CBHW071332150726
47997CB00002B/692